W9-CAU-566

ROSACEA

YOUR SELF-HELP GUIDE

ARLEN BROWNSTEIN, M.S., N.D.
DONNA SHOEMAKER, C.N.
Foreword by Sean O'Laoire, Ph.D.

HARBINGER PUBLICATIONS, INC.

Publisher's Note

Care has been taken to confirm the accuracy of the information presented and to describe generally accepted practices. However, the authors, editors, and publisher are not responsible for errors or omissions or for any consequences from application of the information in this book and make no warranty, express or implied, with respect to the contents of the publication.

The authors, editors, and publisher have exerted every effort to ensure that any drug selection and dosage set forth in this text are in accordance with current recommendations and practice at the time of publication. However, in view of ongoing research, changes in government regulations, and the constant flow of information relating to drug therapy and drug reactions, the reader is urged to check the package insert for each drug for any change in indications and dosage and for added warnings and precautions. This is particularly important when the recommended agent is a new or infrequently employed drug.

Some drugs and medical devices presented in this publication may have Food and Drug Administration (FDA) clearance for limited use in restricted research settings. It is the responsibility of the health care provider to ascertain the FDA status of each drug or device planned for use in their clinical practice.

Distributed in the U.S.A. by Publishers Group West; in Canada by Raincoast Books; in Great Britain by Airlift Book Company, Ltd.; in South Africa by Real Books, Ltd.; in Australia by Boobook; and in New Zealand by Tandem Press.

Copyright © 2001 by Arlen Brownstein and Donna Shoemaker
New Harbinger Publications, Inc.
5674 Shattuck Avenue
Oakland, CA 94609

Cover design © 2001 Lightbourne Images
Text design by Tracy Marie Powell

Library of Congress Card Catalog Number: 00-134867
ISBN 1-57224-224-8 Paperback

All Rights Reserved

Printed in the United States of America

New Harbinger Publications' Web site address: www.newharbinger.com

03   02   01

10   9   8   7   6   5   4   3

Contents

Acknowledgments

I would like to acknowledge Catharine Sutker, who conceived the idea of a book on rosacea and decided that I was the one to write it. I thank Abro Sutker, who, in his own unique style, encouraged me to make this happen. And I am grateful to Heather Garnos, our editor at New Harbinger, for her many helpful suggestions.

My friend Harry Willis contributed the appendix, "Insurance Coverage for Rosacea Treatments." But even more importantly, knowing my aversion to sitting at a desk, he designed the "patented bed desk" for me so I could write in total comfort in my favorite spot. I'm convinced that without it, no book would have been written.

Sean O'Laoire was especially invaluable in the process of creating this book. My ideas on dealing with stress and rosacea come directly from our conversations, and he, alone, is responsible for the chapter called "The Psychology of Face." I very much appreciate his help.

In particular, I would like to thank my parents, Anne and Itz Brownstein, and my brother, Larry Brownstein, whose constant love and support have provided me with a life full of possibilities.
—Arlen Brownstein

I'd like to acknowledge:

Arlen, for getting me into this in the first place, and believing I could do it.

Pamela Strong for her support and insights, and for her meticulous and thorough efforts in helping me ferret out what seemed like countless references.

Kathleen, my loving friend and confidant, whose deep faith in me, and whose respect for my work, are gifts beyond measure.

My family: my parents, David and Eleanor Shoemaker, whose unfailing love, support, and encouragement have carried me beyond what I ever believed I could do; my sister, Sandy, and my brother, Dave, who both knew I could.

My daughter, Buffy, who suffered through years of uninvited nutritional advice, and managed to come through it all, giving me her love and trust (and her bedroom so I could set up an office).

Bill, who believed in me.

Wonderful friends and clients, who have generously given their support, respect, and helpful feedback, so that I can continually improve my efforts.

—Donna Shoemaker

Foreword

Hey, what did I know? Some people are skinny, some are fat, some are tall, some are short, and some are red-faced. That was the natural course of things, or so I thought. Rosacea? Never heard of it! And yet growing up in Ireland, I was surrounded by people with rosacea; it is most common among Celts. It was so common, in fact, that I didn't recognize it as something out of the ordinary. So if it's not a problem, why fix it? Because it *is* a problem, for those who have it, even when others don't recognize it as a disease.

Wearing your disease on your face is very difficult; there is no place to hide. And that has a very significant effect on the psyche. It gets even worse because it becomes a vicious circle: You have a red face to begin with, so you are embarrassed in public situations; embarrassment is a powerful trigger for blushing, which further exacerbates the situation, so your face gets redder—and the cycle continues.

I have known Dr. Brownstein since she first manifested this disease. She tried it all, from herbs to antibiotics. It was all to no avail. There was very little the conventional or alternative medical community could tell her about the disease and even less they could do for her. I watched her process that realization—denial, anger, fear, even panic. It was an awful thought that a beautiful woman might be facing (no pun intended) the possibility of " disfigurement." The good news (to jump ahead to the end of the story and the strength of this book) is that that never happened. But she didn't know that at the beginning. So I watched her anxieties increase as all of her allopathic, homeopathic, and naturopathic options came to naught. The horrible truth was: Nobody knew the cause of rosacea or how to treat it. That was the darkest hour. But as the old saying has it, the darkest hour comes just before the dawn. Arlen invented this particular dawn. And that is what this book is about.

The first faint hint of the coming day was the realization that this was an incurable disease about which nobody but herself could do anything. She began to take control and reframe the issues and turn her rosacea around. That is the great strength of this book. Arlen is not some pedantic researcher, nor some cerebral medic dealing theoretically with an illness they've never had—this book is, in part, the offspring of her own safari through the territory of rosacea. She has walked this talk; what she has to say is practical, and it works.

Dr. Brownstein began to gather information, both from written material, such as it was, and from attending carefully to her own experience. With great care she began to figure out what the triggers were, major and minor. These came from behavior (e.g. strenuous exercise), climate (e.g. sunshine), diet (e.g. spices), and a host of other factors. Understanding her own body and its reactions to inner and outer stimuli became her modus operandi. On a trial and error basis, she built up a repertory of dos and don'ts; a glossary of what helped and what hindered. Slowly but surely she was taking back the reins—embracing the new possibilities rather than bemoaning the old losses.

When it was suggested to her that she write a book on rosacea, she knew, immediately, who should write the nutrition sections. Donna Shoemaker is a dedicated and committed practitioner who manages to stay on the cutting edge of nutritional knowledge. She has proven to be the ideal choice, as will be evident from the chapters she authored. "Thorough" and "competent" are words that come to mind when you read her work. I've also had the privilege of knowing Donna for many years. She is a perfectionist; it shows in all she does, and it shows in her contributions to this book.

Dr. Brownstein comes well-equipped for the task of masterminding the planning of this book. Blessed with a photographic memory and the ability to speed-read, she can distill the essence of a piece of writing very quickly. Thus, for the last nine years, she was able to devour anything that was in print on the topic of rosacea. Books, journals, brochures, and the Internet were vacuumed until they had delivered any and all relevant information. Some people have a great ability to hold a lot of information in their heads. However, it is a totally different gift to be able to synthesize such data, identify patterns there, and present a synopsis that is clear, interesting, and comprehensive. Arlen has that gift, also. And apart from some tongue-twisting, jaw-breaking, multisyllabic, Latin-generated names of medications, she has managed to keep this book simple. Quite a feat!

Having done an exhaustive literature review, and having culled all that was of value, she realized that there was nothing available that wasn't primarily of purely scientific interest. There was nothing for either the practitioner who had run out of options, nor for the suffering layperson for whom the standard protocols had failed. There were no alternatives in the journals. So the authors have trodden a path all of their own making. It wasn't even "the road less traveled." This was pure virgin tundra, with not a semblance of even yak tracks. The result is a compassionate, courageous, humorous, and altogether original book that contains between its covers the complete guide to recognizing and dealing with all facets of the disease.

Obviously, its main audience will be people with rosacea, as well as physicians and health care workers. But it will also speak to family and friends who want to try to support those who suffer. There will, however, be a third benefit, and that is the dismantling of a prejudice—the psychologically crushing stereotypes attributing rosacea symptoms to excessive alcohol consumption. The twentieth century has seen a great number of biases, prejudices, and stereotypes be identified, deconstructed, and dissolved (e.g. racism, sexism, ageism.) Prejudice around disease has been a subcategory all in its own right. In the early part of the century, tuberculosis was an embarrassing thing; families tried to hide it, even as members died of it, and popular "wisdom" nodded its head sagely and winked knowingly. Mental disorders were tagged as shameful and taken as evidence of personal and familial weakness. Cancer patients were often asked, "What have you done to cause this illness?" Then AIDS was seen as a divine retribution for lifestyles some considered "depraved."

Gratefully, in each instance, intelligent and compassionate people stepped up to the plate and began to study these diseases, helping both the sufferers and the healthy—and, most importantly of all, re-educating the whole culture so that animosity and fear gave way to understanding and acceptance. This book is in such a tradition. It will do much to vaporize the negative, judgmental myths surrounding rosacea.

This book was written because there was nothing worthwhile out there. Dr. Brownstein is speaking from and writing for an underserved and underrecognized population.

Models of reality allow us to navigate in the real world, but all models of reality are approximations. This is especially true in the medical world—and so, diagnosis, treatment, and prognosis are not watertight. The authors of this book are aware of this. That's why they have given us lots of useful and practical information and suggestions for dealing with a model of rosacea, which will hold true a lot of the time. But recognizing that each individual is unique and may experience rosacea in an idiosyncratic fashion, they have included many tips that will allow you to gauge and respond to *your* experience of the disease. They have included exercises that will allow you to gather your own data, identify patterns in it, and respond specifically to what works for you.

If you are interested in a *"How come . . . ?"* book on understanding rosacea, this is the one. If what you want is a *"How to . . . ?"* manual for dealing with the disease, you won't find anything that even remotely touches this book for quality and practical wisdom.

You got the disease? You got this book? You just got lucky!

—Sean O'Laoire

Introduction

by Arlen Brownstein, N.D.

Not everything that is faced can be changed,
but nothing can be changed until it is faced.

—James Baldwin

I always thought I was destined to have beautiful skin as I aged, because I was born with a secret weapon: I hated the sun. As a teenager, I ruined many a beach day for my friends as I beseeched after less than an hour, "Is it time to leave yet?" My friend Barb used to tell everyone that she had a friend who was going to look great when she was forty. Of course, the implication was that for a seventeen-year-old, lily white was not the most desirable look.

In the 1960s, most people didn't know or didn't believe that the sun could irreparably damage the skin. Worse yet, there were no chemical sunscreens on the market, and it seemed like everyone was using baby oil instead. My guess is the goal was to intensify the baking process, otherwise known as tanning.

In my twenties and thirties, my dislike for the sun grew stronger. I always joked that it was my kryptonite, weakening me the same way that fragments from the planet Krypton affected Superman. There were a lot of activities that I didn't share in with my friends, but I was comforted by the knowledge that at least I had lovely skin and would for many decades. There'd be no wrinkles or leathery skin for me.

Then my forties hit, and I soon found myself in early menopause. Looking back, it's clear to me that my rosacea first appeared at that time. Two incidents stand out in my mind. The first occasion was a hike with friends on a hot day. This is something I was always loath to do, but I found myself in a social situation where it was impossible to bow out. The walk lasted too long, because we got lost in the Marin hills. When we got back home, I was shocked to see my face. It was beet red and stayed that way for hours. The second incident took place at a Passover Seder where I had consumed a small amount of wine. Someone said something that I found slightly embarrassing and I blushed to such an extreme degree that everyone started laughing at me. I remember thinking that my overreaction was peculiar.

At the same time, something else was happening. I had always been sensitive to skin products, but now it seemed like everything irritated my skin. More often than not, a face cream or cleanser made my skin burn. And after I washed my face, my skin felt very tight, as if the cleanser hadn't been completely removed. I hated the sensation and I found myself going back to rinse my face over and over and over again. Yet I still didn't get that something was going on with my skin.

Then came the next stage, and it wasn't pretty. My face, which had always been unblemished, started to break out. Was it acne or a rash? I couldn't figure out what was going on, but I soon came up with an idea: It must have something to do with my cats. For years I had been violently allergic to them with all the manifestations of a respiratory allergy: the constant sneezing and the runny, itchy eyes. Then through natural medicine, primarily homeopathy, I had become allergy free. Now I was living a blissfully sneeze-free life with four cats, all of whom slept on my bed or in close proximity, depending on their mood. (I had bought a king-size bed so there was room for everyone, including my dog, Remedy.) What was happening, I concluded, was that although my respiratory allergies were gone, I was now manifesting symptoms on my skin instead. So I figured that what I had was simply a contact dermatitis, and all I needed to do was keep cat fur off my face in order to get my flawless complexion back. I had a two-pronged approach to this goal. First, I changed bedrooms, causing great consternation to my cat Shaina, who had been sleeping with me for almost fifteen years. Second, whenever I was in the house, I'd cover my face with a scarf. My husband told me I was crazy and looked ridiculous. He was right on both counts, but I was desperate to figure out what was going on. It didn't take long to realize that my brilliant idea wasn't so brilliant and that I wasn't going to solve the problem this way. And besides, it was really hot and uncomfortable under that scarf.

Now remember, I'm a trained naturopathic physician—and yet I was walking around the house with a bandanna covering everything but my eyes. The lesson I learned from this is that panic sets in when something affects your face. You do silly things, because you act out of fear and embarrassment.

I had studied dermatology, and all my friends were connected in some way with the health field. Yet no one recognized what I had, despite the fact that it was literally staring us in the face. We had all been taught about rosacea, and then promptly forgot about it. It was not given a lot of emphasis in our education. How could that be? Why is there so little knowledge about a disorder that affects millions of people?

The truth is that I secretly had a much greater fear, and that's where my mind was focused. Seeing that rash across my cheeks, my mind immediately went to lupus, a serious autoimmune disorder. When you study medicine, and you have a tendency toward hypochondriasis, you're in a lot of trouble. At school I was sure I had every fatal disease, so naturally the blotches on my face would cause me to jump to the worst-case scenario.

And of course, the worry caused its own problems. As those of you know who already have rosacea, and as the rest of you will learn who are new to this disorder, worry is stressful, and stress is the main trigger for the symptoms of rosacea. I was afraid now of what I might have and it really scared me that I couldn't seem to get control of it. I was trying many types of natural treatments, but nothing was really working. The truth is that I definitely should not have been treating myself, because in my distress with my worsening appearance, I was not thinking things out logically and unemotionally like I would have been able to do for someone else.

I did, however, eventually have the sense to have blood work done and could put my fears of lupus to rest. With that off my mind, I was then able to think more sensibly, and finally realized that it had to be rosacea. It seemed strange: I had no knowledge of any family history, and no one else in my immediate family had been affected. Ethnically, I didn't fit the typical profile, though I did have unusually light skin. I also wondered why I'd never known anyone who had it, considering that it's such a common disorder. Or had I? Before I had rosacea, I never noticed the symptoms on anyone. Now there's barely a day that goes by that I don't see it. As I've educated my friends, they tell me the same thing. They see it constantly, and they've probably seen it all their lives. It's not some new disease—in fact, it was first described medically as early as the fourteenth century. Early literature, such as Shakespeare's *Henry V*, depicts red-faced men with large, bulbous noses. And throughout the centuries, artists have painted this same look, the look of advanced rosacea.

I did go to a dermatologist to confirm my diagnosis. There was no doubt in his mind that I had rosacea. Then, in desperate straits and in direct opposition to my training and belief in natural medicine, I began the prescribed medical program. It worked for a short while, and then it stopped. I applied an assortment of topical ointments, to no avail and sometimes even to the detriment of my skin. Different dermatologists were tried and abandoned. I became obsessed with the state of my face, checking my skin constantly. Fortunately, I had reached the stage of life where my close vision was awful, so I couldn't see much. Unfortunately, I started needing a magnifying mirror, so then all my imperfections were grossly exaggerated.

Finally, I came to my senses and realized that I had the tools and the knowledge to approach rosacea naturally and to get good results. I began taking nutrients to strengthen my capillaries. I took great care to consume the essential fatty acids that would activate the anti-inflammatory pathways in my body. I took digestive enzymes with every meal. I started paying very close attention to what I put into my body, so I could identify my triggers. Even a sip of wine would cause me to wake up the next morning with a red blotch on my face. But the most painful thing of all was the knowledge that my days of a nice piece of chocolate cake, my favorite indulgence, were over. Chocolate causes an aggravation for me that can literally last months.

Although the appearance of my face improved dramatically, I was still left with dilated capillaries on my cheeks and nose. I have undergone laser treatments and light therapies a number of times and these have helped enormously. I am grateful that I had the opportunity to avail myself of these treatments. However, during the procedure, when I'm very uncomfortable (it feels like a rubber band being snapped against your face), I still curse the fates that made this necessary.

I never had a chronic disease before rosacea, so I couldn't begin to know how it might consume my life. Because of its very nature, it constantly makes itself known. But I've made my peace with it, and so can you. I may never be able to forget that I have it, but truthfully, it's lost its power to control me. The charge just isn't there anymore. Oh, I still complain about having it, but emotionally it no longer causes me pain. I may see a group of my friends drinking wine and think longingly that it would be nice to have a glass also, but that's about it. Vegetarians may feel the same way when they see their friends eating the Thanksgiving turkey. Everybody has something he or she can't do.

If you have had rosacea for a while, your story is probably pretty much like mine: the initial puzzlement at the symptoms, then disbelief, and finally dismay, embarrassment, sometimes even depression. Through trial and error and probably your own research and experimentation, you may have hit upon a program that works for you. We hope this book will give you more ideas to incorporate into your self-treatment.

For those of you who are new to this disorder or just beginning to realize what is happening to your skin, our goal is to save you the frustrating years that many of us have had to go through pretty much on our own. The earlier you work on controlling your rosacea, the easier it is to deal with.

We make no judgments about how you decide to treat your rosacea. This disease is too complicated and frustrating to say there is only one way to approach it. If you are someone who is satisfied with the standard medical approach and it's working for you, then that's the right way for you to go. However, if you are someone who has tried the conventional route with no success, or someone who prefers to face rosacea without a lifetime of medication, then the more natural approach is what you need to explore. For me personally, the naturopathic approach, which treats the whole body and not just the disease, makes the most sense.

You will notice the emphasis on nutrition in this book. The reason is simple. We believe that eating right, taking appropriate supplements, and optimizing your digestive system can improve your rosacea, not to mention your overall health. Whether you make a good nutritional program the core of your treatment, or whether you treat it as an adjunct to conventional medical treatment, you will benefit greatly.

This book is primarily for those for whom rosacea is a cosmetic disorder. That is to say, there is a disease process that is showing up on your face that makes you self-conscious and is emotionally distressing. There may occasionally be some burning or itching, but if you didn't have a mirror, most of the time you'd be feeling just fine. The majority of people who have rosacea fall into this category. There is, however, a subset of people who suffer to a much greater degree. They may have severe burning and throbbing pains in their face, and the quality of their life is affected, whether or not they have access to a mirror. If you are one of these people, there is definitely useful information for you in this book and you will benefit, but please understand that this book is geared toward the more common manifestations of rosacea.

For me, finally accepting how common rosacea is was actually very helpful. It's somehow comforting seeing all these strangers around me coping with the same experience in their lives. It's like all of us having the same unusual eye color or belonging to the same club, our own Rosacean Society. Not too long ago I was eating in a restaurant and I said to my dinner companion, "See that woman over there, she has rosacea." And then I laughed. "Wouldn't it be funny if she were saying to her friend, 'See that woman over there, she has rosacea.'" The next step will be for me to actually say to someone's face, "I see you have rosacea, so do I." If we can all stop being so self-conscious about what has been called "the embarrassing disease," the emotional distress over this disorder will decrease enormously. Rosaceans of the world: Let's unite and work on it.

Visit "Rosacea World," the Web site

My determination to overcome rosacea and its effects on my life inspired me to write this book and to share with others the benefit of my own thoughts and research. Further, to continue where this book leaves off, and to provide dynamic, interactive support that the printed page simply cannot, I have built a Web site called "Rosacea World" (www.rosaceaworld.com), the mission of which is to provide a gathering place. I encourage you to visit the site for recent developments in rosacea, to ask questions about the latest in research and treatment, and to share your thoughts and feelings about your own experience.

I

What Is Rosacea?

Rosacea is a chronic skin disorder that results in facial flushing, dilated capillaries, acneiform lesions, and swelling, among other symptoms. In many cases, rosacea also affects the eyes. It may be hard to imagine, especially if you feel no one around you understands what you're going through, but this disorder is actually fairly common, with an estimated thirteen million or more affected people in the United States alone. That's at least one out of twenty people (National Rosacea Society 1998). Worldwide, it affects tens of millions. It's amazing when you think about it: 5 percent of Americans have this disorder, and yet almost 80 percent of us, according to surveys, have never even heard of it. The truth is, people see it all the time, but they don't recognize it for what it is. Even people who have rosacea often don't realize what they have.

What Does Rosacea Look Like?

It starts innocently enough—so innocently, in fact, that it is seldom recognized. After all, would you consider excessive blushing the beginning of a disease? Would you be alarmed if your face turned red after being in the sun or exposed to the wind? And honestly, would you think there was something amiss if you flushed after a glass or two of wine?

That is why rosacea is so hard to recognize in its earliest stages. The changes to your face are gradual, until one day you realize that something is clearly wrong. Maybe the redness that was once an occasional flush seems much more frequent, or perhaps it is now always present. You may notice that your skin feels dry or like it's pulled tight against your skull. Or you may notice that your face looks shiny or oily. On further inspection, it may seem that your pores, especially on your nose, have gotten much larger. And to top it all off, you have what appears to be acne, perhaps for the first time in your life.

At this point, vanity would most likely direct you to your health care provider or to a dermatologist, who would probably be able to diagnose your changing complexion as rosacea.

Rosacea is a disease with two components that are connected in some mysterious way that is not yet understood. The first part is vascular, meaning it has to do with blood vessels. People with rosacea have an abnormality of the facial blood vessels that causes excessive flushing. This flushing is most common across the blush areas of the face—cheeks, chin, forehead, and nose. Occasionally, the neck and upper chest will also be affected Symptoms are episodic in nature, and may seem at times to appear or disappear randomly. These symptoms can manifest as overall flushing or as individual blotches. Initially, the flushing is occasional, but when it becomes more frequent, it leads to red lines on the face, dilated capillaries, that don't go away. These thin, red lines are called *telangiectasia*.

The second component of rosacea is an inflammatory reaction of the sebaceaous (oil) glands of your face. It is believed that this is the result of the flushing, but how or why this happens is, you guessed it, another mystery. What *is* known is that this inflammatory response causes the acne of rosacea, which appears as two different types of lesions—papules and pustules. Papules are small, red, elevated and solid; pustules are pus-filled. This type of acne differs from acne vulgaris, or teenage acne, through an absence of comedones, more commonly known as blackheads and whiteheads.

Just because you have rosacea doesn't mean that you will have all the symptoms that are associated with the disease. Some people have only the acne-type lesions. Others have just generalized flushing. Someone else may suffer from a bright red nose. A person with a combination of symptoms often experiences one of the symptoms to a greater extent.

Differences Between the Sexes

It should be noted that men and women tend to have different problem areas. Women are more likely to have symptoms on their cheeks and chin. The forehead seems to be affected almost equally in men and women. However, probably the most unfortunate symptom of rosacea, *rhinophyma*, occurs much more frequently in men. Rhinophyma is an abnormal growth of the tissue of the nose. There have been different theories to account for this advanced-stage development, but the latest research attributes it to the chronic swelling, or *lymphadema*, that can occur with rosacea (Aloi et al. 2000). Flushing leads to the accumulation of fluid under the skin. Because the lymphatic system cannot clear it quickly or adequately enough, chronic changes occur that lead to the buildup of excess tissue.

With rhinophyma, small bumps appear on the nose, which eventually becomes large and bulbous, often with a reddish-purple coloration. Imagine W. C. Fields and you get the picture. This is the symptom that the general public notices most often, yet most people don't realize that it's entirely due to rosacea. Unfortunately, it's generally assumed to be a sign of excess alcohol consumption.

Rhinophyma isn't the only result of lymphadema. The excess fluid under the top layer of skin can also cause the face to swell. For some people, this symptom occurs relatively early in the course of rosacea. Again, it is the flushing that causes fluid to build up in the tissues of the face. This extra fluid can cause the cheeks to have a baggy appearance and may lead to the development of excess tissue on the face and nose. The swelling is minimal or unnoticeable for some, and uncomfortable and even painful for others.

What Does Rosacea Feel Like?

Most rosaceans have no pain at all, while others feel pain ranging from mild to severe. Rosacea sometimes causes the skin to itch, and it may also cause a burning sensation that ranges from mild to intense. Among those with more severe cases resulting in pain in the inflamed areas, some even have throbbing, debilitating pain.

Ocular Rosacea

It is very important to recognize that at least 50 percent of people with rosacea experience symptoms involving the eyes (Jenkins et al. 1980). This condition is known as ocular rosacea, and, surprisingly, it may even precede skin symptoms. In fact, it's estimated that about 20 percent of people experience eye symptoms before they ever have skin symptoms (Borrie 1953). For most people, the symptoms are mild, and they don't pose any threat to vision. Perhaps you'll experience a little burning or notice a slight redness to your eyes. You may notice that they have become sensitive to light, or maybe they even feel gritty or like there is a foreign body in them.

It is not uncommon for people with rosacea to have chronic inflammation of the margins of the eyelids, which is called *blepharitis*. There are two types: one causes tiny ulcers at the lid margins, and the other causes greasy flaking on the eyelashes. Another very common problem is sties, which occur when there is an infection of the eyelash follicles. Sties are often a direct result of blepharitis. A small, inflamed, painful pustule appears on the lid margin and then eventually resolves on its own. Sties are very common in people with rosacea; many ophthalmologists believe that the majority of people who get sties will eventually go on to develop rosacea.

There is also *meibomian gland* involvement in ocular rosacea. These are small glands on the margins of the eyelids whose job is to lubricate the lids by producing a fatty secretion that enables them to move easily over the surface of the eye. The oily layer produced by the meibomian glands also reduces evaporation of tears. If an acute inflammation of one of these glands occurs, you get an internal sty. You may also develop a *chalazion*, which is an enlargement of a meibomian gland resulting from it being plugged up and inflamed. Most will disappear on their own after a few months, although some will require removal by a physician. Other symptoms that are not uncommon to the eyelids are telangiectasia, swelling, and loss of eyelashes.

Much rarer, but not unheard of, is corneal involvement, where sight can actually be threatened. Expect your eye symptoms to be minor if you have them at all, but be aware that there is always the potential for something more serious to occur. So, if your eyes are really bothering you, take charge and go see an ophthalmologist for an evaluation. For some unknown reason, especially considering the common occurrence of eye symptoms with rosacea, it is very unusual for a dermatologist to even bring up the subject.

Eve, a massage therapist, says, "I consider it absolutely amazing that, in the past ten years since I developed rosacea, I have seen at least three different dermatologists and not one of them ever even asked me if my eyes were bothering me. And they were! I had constant burning and the sense that something was floating around in my eye that didn't belong there. My poor husband was constantly searching for an eyelash in my eye that wasn't there. I just never connected the eyes with the rosacea, and so I didn't know it could be treated. It seems that so many of the problems with rosacea you have to figure out on your own and then manage yourself."

Individual Symptoms

If you have rosacea, you're already aware of the myriad possible symptoms. And yet there may be even more than the ones discussed here. Some rosaceans are convinced that they have additional symptoms, albeit out of the norm, that are connected to the disease. They are frustrated because their doctors won't address these symptoms, either because they don't believe they exist, or more likely, because they don't know what to do with them. Find a doctor who will listen to you and who understands that each individual manifests symptoms in their own unique way.

What old-timers know and newcomers will discover is that rosacea, for the vast majority of us, doesn't simply go away by itself. Initially, it may appear to do just that, going into remission for periods of time. But it will reappear, and you must be prepared to address it with either conventional or alternative treatments. You can use a list like the one on the next page to track your symptoms.

You Can't Pass It On
(Except Hereditarily)

In case you or anyone close to you is concerned, it is important to understand that rosacea is not contagious. It can *not* be passed on to anyone else by contact or inhalation, nor can you spread it yourself from one area of your face to another. Although antibiotics are a common treatment, they are used for their anti-inflammatory action, not because rosacea is an infectious disease.

Rosacea Symptoms

❋ Flushing, primarily of the blush areas of the face

❋ Increased shiny appearance to the face

❋ Feeling of or actual dryness of the face

❋ Telangiectasia

❋ Blemishes (papules and pustules)

❋ Increased pore size

❋ Swelling of the face, especially the nose

❋ Eye involvement (eyelid inflammation, conjunctivitis, keratitis, sensitivity to sunlight)

❋ Hyperirritability of the skin to cosmetics, creams, sunscreens, etc.

❋ Burning and tingling of the skin

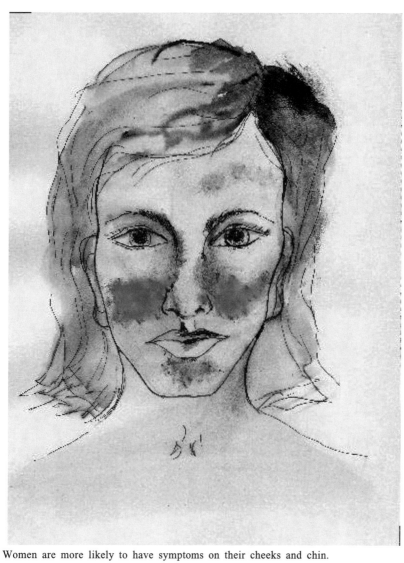

Women are more likely to have symptoms on their cheeks and chin.

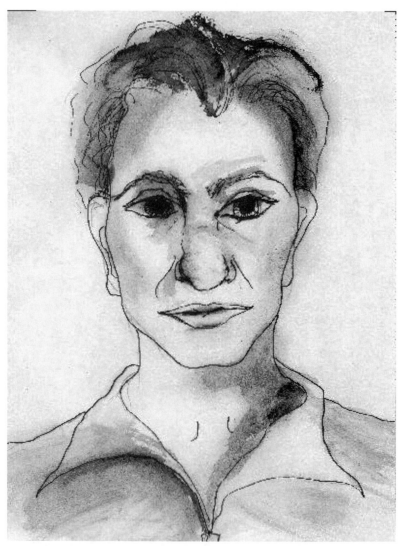

Rhinophyma, an abnormal growth of the tissue of the nose, occurs much more frequently in men.

2

Rosacea Basics

What Causes Rosacea?

Just about everything concerning rosacea is a puzzle, including its cause. There are plenty of hypotheses, but nothing has yet been proven. "Perhaps nowhere else in dermatology is so little known about a condition that affects so many," says Dr. Jonathan Wilkin, chairman of the medical advisory board for the National Rosacea Society's research grants program. Proposed etiologies have included infectious agents, immune disorders, hyperactive sebaceous glands, and gastrointestinal bacteria called *helicobacter pylori*. One of the latest ideas making the rounds has to do with the *demodex folliculorum* mite that lives on human skin. The thought here is that these mites burrow into facial follicles, clog up oil glands, and cause inflammation. While it's true that rosacea sufferers seem to have more of these mites on their skin, some researchers contend that they take up residence there because the skin is already inflamed.

Another theory being considered is that because of a breakdown in connective tissue, small blood vessels are not being supported adequately, which in turn leads to prolonged vasodilation. There also appears to be some change in the skin, a thinning, that makes the capillaries (and thus the flushing) more visible. But again the question is: What could cause these things to happen? Is it simply an unfortunate combination of genetics and environment?

There is no hypothesis, as of yet, that can explain why rosacea includes both vascular and inflammatory reactions. The only thing known for sure, through observation, is that rosacea is related to how often and how strongly people flush. This is leading more and more people to believe that rosacea is primarily a vascular disorder. Somehow this rosiness leads to all of the major symptoms: the red face, the swelling, the telangiectasia, and the papules and pustules. There is speculation that the flushing may somehow be connected to a nervous system defect; along these lines, it is interesting to note that the worst rosacea flare-ups occur during stressful situations.

It would be nice to pinpoint the exact cause of rosacea and why the switch is turned on for some people but not others. But, because the cause of rosacea is unknown at this time, you must accept the fact that the various treatments are based solely on what has been seen to help others with the disorder. Often it's not known why something works, but don't let that worry you. Rosacea is a complex disorder that may develop for different reasons in different people. It's unlikely that researchers will ever arrive at an explanation that fits all cases.

Is It Really Rosacea?

There are no diagnostic tests for rosacea, except for a punch biopsy, which is very seldom done. Instead, the diagnosis is based entirely on clinical findings: That is, your skin is usually the giveaway. However, even if it seems obvious to you that you have rosacea, you shouldn't self-diagnose, because there are other disorders that can be mistaken for rosacea. See a dermatologist or other knowledgeable health care provider so you can be sure what it is you actually have and that you're treating it appropriately. He or she will examine the lesions on your face, taking note of their color, size, and pattern. Some conditions that may look similar to rosacea are adult acne, allergic dermatitis, seborrheic dermatitis, perioral dermatitis, lupus erythematosus, and iatrogenic (treatment-induced) rosacea.

    ❀ **Acne** can be ruled out if there are whiteheads and blackheads and the pimples cover the whole face instead of just the blush areas. Acne lesions are also common on the chest, neck, and upper back.

❋ **Allergic dermatitis** occurs when something that comes in contact with your skin causes symptoms such as itching or a chronic rash. Perhaps you're reacting to your makeup or to a cat rubbing against your face. You can even become reactive to medicines or cosmetics you have used topically for years.

❋ **Seborrheic dermatitis** is an inflammatory scaling disease. It generally appears on the scalp, and, when more severe, on the face and other parts of the body. In its milder form, it is simply dandruff. If it becomes more severe, scaling papules can appear on the face. Sometimes it is difficult to distinguish this condition from rosacea, and to make it more confusing, it's not unusual for an individual to have both simultaneously.

❋ **Perioral dermatitis** appears as an eruption of pimples and bumps around the mouth and on the chin. It is found predominantly in women and may occur concurrently with rosacea.

❋ **Lupus erythematosus** presents with a rash that looks like a butterfly across the central portion of the face. Unlike rosacea, the rash is scaly. The lesions are usually flat, red areas, and there are no pustules. This can be a very serious illness and must be ruled out. Fortunately, it can be diagnosed with blood work.

❋ **Iatrogenic (treatment induced) rosacea** is caused by prolonged use of a corticosteroid ointment. As a result, the skin becomes thin and fragile, and the capillary walls are weakened. The walls then rupture and cause the face to flush. Think twice before you put cortisone cream on your face for any reason: It's not worth the short-term benefit of cosmetic improvement, because it will ultimately be harmful to the appearance of your skin.

Even dermatologists can't always be sure if it's rosacea simply by looking at you—and they see it all the time. But it's still important to get a diagnosis, because if you self-diagnose and you're wrong, you could be in trouble. You certainly don't want to overlook a more serious illness that might require treatment. On the flip side, if you mistakenly decide that what you have isn't rosacea and self-treat for some other condition instead, you could easily worsen the rosacea. For example, products made for acne can cause a terrible flare-up in someone with rosacea. It's best to get a diagnosis. After that, your approach to treatment is up to you.

Who Is Most at Risk?

The causes of rosacea are still mysterious, but we do know a few things about which populations are most likely to get it.

It's in the Genes

There appears to be a hereditary link to this chronic skin condition. A 1999 survey by the National Rosacea Society indicated that nearly 40 percent of the 2,052 respondents had a family member who also had rosacea. It is widely believed that rosacea affects mainly fair-skinned people of Celtic or northern European descent. In fact, it has often been called the "Curse of the Celts," although the English have a rate of rosacea not far behind the Irish. Other groups with an elevated incidence of rosacea are those of Lithuanian, Polish, Balkan, and Scandinavian descent.

Although the vast majority of people with rosacea have light skin, darker-skinned people sometimes get rosacea too. It may be that increased pigmentation in African-Americans, Hispanics, and Asians may be masking rosacea, and the symptoms of the disease are just more obvious in lighter-skinned individuals. Or it may be that having darker skin is somehow naturally protective against rosacea.

For African-Americans, the symptoms of rosacea will differ somewhat from those of lighter-skinned individuals. The redness will have a violet hue, and although flushing can not be seen, they will report a definite sense of warmth in rosacea blush areas. Papules and pustules and the increased oiliness of the face are also possible manifestations. An added problem they may encounter is hyperpigmentation, a darkening of the areas of the face where inflammation has occurred.

Age Matters

Rosacea is most prevalent in people in their thirties to fifties, although it is said that anyone past puberty is a candidate. And while the medical texts don't generally recognize rosacea occurring in children, there are people who believe they have had the disease since childhood, based on their memories of being ridiculed for their bright red noses.

The Sober Truth

There is a common misconception that links rosacea to alcoholism. (You'll remember our earlier discussion of rhinophyma, which many people mistakenly believe is a sign of excessive drinking.) Drinking can, indeed, make rosacea worse, but it doesn't cause it. Many people who never drink have rosacea, and many people who drink excessively never get it.

Gender Issues

It is now thought that women are affected with rosacea considerably more often than men. However, men seem to have more severe symptoms, although it may simply be that the symptoms are more severe, because, as with most ailments, men tend to put off seeing a health professional as long as possible. It is not unusual to find that for some women, the onset seems to be associated with menopause. It is intriguing to ponder why the hot flashes of menopause may lead to rosacea for some women, but not others.

Blushing Turns to Flushing

A feature common to most people who get rosacea is a history of blushing easily. The adolescent who has a charming peaches and cream complexion and blushes at the drop of a hat is often a prime candidate to develop the disorder as she or he gets older.

Many women with rosacea remember having had especially lovely skin. Sheila, a receptionist, is not unusual when she says, "I was always proud of my porcelain complexion and got lots of compliments. I didn't even have any problems as a teenager. I was a blusher, but I was told it was charming, so I didn't mind."

So Sensitive

Another early warning indicator is a history of hyperreactive skin. you may be one of those people who often reacted adversely to things you put on your face. Soaps would make your skin burn, creams would cause rashes and products would be tried and discarded.

Kayla, a physician of Russian Jewish background, illustrates how puzzling rosacea can be. She seems to be the only person in her family to have the disease and she doesn't fit the common ethnic profile. "I was shocked and still am. I keep wondering where it came from, although, thinking back, I wonder if my grandmother had ocular rosacea. She was always complaining that her eyes hurt, burned terribly. Maybe she just didn't manifest any skin symptoms. Or maybe she did and no one noticed, because her skin was very dark. As for me, although many of my relative are dark, I am incredibly light-skinned. In addition, I have a long history of reacting to facial products. I've always thought of myself as having sensitive skin."

Knowing of a hereditary component to rosacea doesn't much help you if you currently have the disorder. However, it may help others in your family to recognize it in its beginning stages when it is easiest to treat. Do them all a huge favor, and educate them about the early warning signs.

3

Treatment Options for Rosacea

How It Begins

If you've already been diagnosed with and treated for rosacea, chances are your experience went a bit like this: You walked into the office of a dermatologist. After taking one look at you, she said, "You have a classic case of rosacea." A short time later, you left the office with a prescription for antibiotics, a prescription for MetroGel, and two pamphlets put out by the National Rosacea Society.

Even if the dermatologist is not completely certain of the diagnosis, the procedure is generally the same, because the doctor knows that if you respond to the antibiotics, rosacea is the best diagnosis. If you don't respond, then other diseases can be considered, and blood tests may be ordered to rule out more serious disorders.

But let's get back again to you walking out of that office. You suddenly find yourself in the disconcerting position of having an illness with no known cause, no known cure, and no information out there for you except the two pamphlets in your hand. And all you know at this point is that you will do anything to get your face back, because, after all, the very reason you're at the doctor's office in the first place is because your skin is out of control.

At this stage, almost everyone, even those devoted to natural medicine, will be tempted to go the standard route. With other disorders, people may be willing to let the cure take time, but there's something about a disease right out there on your face that makes you want to suppress the symptoms immediately.

Oral Medications

For most people, the antibiotics do provide relief from symptoms within a week or two. Some of these people find that the therapy works for them in the long term, and they stay on it. For others, the initial treatment stops working and they begin the cycle of trying all kinds of different medications. A number of different broad-spectrum antibiotics are prescribed for rosacea, primarily tetracycline and sometimes minocycline or doxycycline. (Keep in mind that antibiotics are used not because rosacea is an infection, but because they seem to help diminish the inflammatory response.) The use of antibiotics is eventually phased out for most people because of the many side effects associated with them, such as chronic yeast infections and gastrointestinal upset. But even some of those people troubled by side effects stay on the drugs indefinitely, because they feel they have no other options; nothing else they've been prescribed seems to work for them.

For severe rosacea that is unresponsive to other drugs, isotretinoin (Accutane) may be prescribed. It is a potent anti-inflammatory, that can reduce the occurrence of papules and pustules and decrease severe, burning pain. But it can also have significant side effects that need to be considered. Accutane can cause severe birth defects, so women of childbearing age need to be very careful of this drug. A common occurrence among Accutane users is extremely chapped, peeling, and sometimes bleeding lips. Burning and dry eyes are another possibility. If you are already dealing with ocular rosacea, you probably don't want to add this to the mix. Question your doctor in depth if this drug is ever prescribed for you, so that you can make an informed decision. There are people who have taken Accutane who feel they benefited enormously, those who feel they got no benefit, and those who feel that the benefit they achieved was not worth the side effects.

There are other oral medications that are used for people who flush severely and uncontrollably. Potent drugs, such as beta-blockers (e.g., propranolol) and alpha-antagonists (e.g., clonidine), are used by people whose social flushing is so devastating that their lives are limited by it. These may be prescribed for rosaceans.

Topical Medications

Topical medications are used either in conjunction with oral medications or by themselves. The most commonly prescribed is metronidazole, which is an antibacterial, antifungal agent. It is used to decrease inflammatory lesions, which you probably know as the breakouts. How it works is really not understood, but it does seem to work very well for some people. Yet others will swear that it makes their rosacea worse. As you'll learn later in the chapter on triggers, each rosacean must find what works and doesn't work for them. Nothing works for everyone. Metronidazole is marketed by different companies, but it is most commonly prescribed in the form of MetroGel and MetroCream— the cream being less drying than the gel. Recently, the company that makes these products came out with MetroLotion, and tests are showing that this may be the most effective of the three. Remember, if you use any topical products, you must apply them to your whole face. It's not like in the days of teenage acne when you applied medication only to the visible blemishes. If you decide to use one of these products, it's important to administer it properly.

If you find yourself in this world of medication, you may end up running the gamut of topical treatments. Your doctor might prescribe topical antibiotics, such as erythromycin, or she might suggest you try Noritate (another metronidazole product, but in a different base), Klaron, or Sulfacet. If you're typical, you'll get to try them all at one time or another. Sometimes physicians, too, are frustrated as they suggest one medication after another, hoping that they'll hit the right one for you. Unfortunately, even if a topical treatment works for a while, there is no guarantee that it will continue to do so.

Another medication that is rarely prescribed, but that works well for some, is azelaic acid. It is a naturally occurring compound that has anti-inflammatory properties. It comes in both prescription and nonprescription forms. The prescription form is marketed under the name Azelex, and the nonprescription is sold by Ecological Formulas. Although they both contain azelaic acid, the formulations of the products are different. Unfortunately, the nonprescription azelaic acid contains alcohol, which may irritate your skin.

Once again, it's important to remember everyone's response to these medications is different. Samantha recounts being very upset because she was having an unusually bad flare-up. "For some reason that I don't understand, the end of November is traditionally a terrible time for my face. I went back on antibiotics, but this time they worked for a few days and stopped. My standard salves weren't working. I went, in panic, to a new dermatologist and he prescribed a sulfur-based cream that is often used for rosacea. I put it on that night, and when I woke up the next morning and looked in the mirror, I totally freaked. I had never looked so awful. I was so blotchy and inflamed that I was embarrassed to go out in public. It was at that point that I realized that for me, personally, the standard treatments were probably not the best way to go."

Check Out Your Options

Samantha is not alone in feeling that the standard medical treatment isn't right for her. There are many different reasons that people come to this decision, the most common being that the oral and topical treatments just aren't working. Or perhaps if the drugs appear to be working on the skin, they are adversely affecting some other part of the body.

A good example of this is the common use of antibiotics in treating rosacea. They may initially help with the skin, but even the most conservative of practitioners these days recognizes the problems and potential danger of long-term antibiotic use. There are many people whose vision of good health care does not allow for the use of antibiotics except in emergency situations. They are also not comfortable continually putting antibacterial and antifungal creams on their face.

So between the people who are not being sufficiently helped by the conventional treatments for rosacea, and those people who are philosophically opposed to that type of treatment, there is a large population constantly searching for answers. Often they are on their own in their quest, their physicians not being able to offer them anything new. It's an awful moment when you realize that your doctor has tried all her tricks and you still have a complexion that makes you self-conscious.

If you are one of those people, realize that you do have other treatment choices, including the many self-care ideas described in this book. You can also consult alternative practitioners, who will approach your rosacea in a very different way. Consider, for example, seeing a naturopathic physician, who will recognize the importance of treating your whole body, not just your face. A naturopath's goal is to strengthen your entire being, not just focus on one particular disorder.

Naturopathy

Naturopathy is a system of medicine based on the concept of *vis medicatrix naturae,* which translates as "the healing power of nature." It began in Europe in the 1800s, where it was termed "the nature cure." When it came to the United States at the turn of the century, it became known as naturopathy. Until the beginning of the twentieth century, naturopathic medicine was a well-known discipline, practiced throughout the country by thousands of practitioners. Then came the advent of more "scientific medicine." Antibiotics and other pharmaceuticals became the miracle drugs, and natural solutions were considered old-fashioned. Naturopathic medicine, with its gentle therapies and belief in the ability of the body to cure itself, went into decline. But it seems the decline was only temporary, because by the 1970s, people began to realize that modern medicine didn't have the cure for everything, certainly not chronic disease. Many people then decided it was time to take back control of their own health care and to seek the advice of alternative practitioners. The timing was perfect for the rebirth of naturopathy in this country. Naturopathic medical schools began reappearing and a new generation of naturopathic physicians began their training. And it's a unique training: Not only are these doctors schooled in conventional medical sciences, but they are also trained extensively in areas such as nutrition, botanical medicine, physical medicine (e.g., spinal manipulation), and counseling. But be aware: There are people who call themselves naturopaths who have only taken mail-order classes or have very limited training. If you see a naturopathic physician, make sure that she or he has graduated from an accredited four-year naturopathic medical school.

A visit to a naturopathic physician may be a very different experience for you. You'll be asked extensive questions about your diet and your lifestyle. The state of your digestion will be questioned and addressed. And instead of leaving with prescription drugs, you will most likely find yourself being advised to change your diet and to take nutritional supplements.

Most naturopaths have very eclectic practices, using a variety of treatments, such as nutrition, botanical medicine, and manipulation. Other naturopaths tend to specialize primarily in homeopathic medicine or Chinese medicine. These are areas of natural medicine that may also be practiced by other types of health care providers. You should know that there are choices of different medical systems outside of standard Western medicine.

Visit to a Naturopathic Physician

Tina, a thirty-five-year-old from Portland, Oregon, was frustrated by her inability to get control of her rosacea. "I didn't have a major problem with flushing. I'm just slightly pink most of the time, but my face was so oily and bumpy looking. I tried everything my dermatologist prescribed for three years, but nothing really worked. The creams all irritated my face and made it worse, and the antibiotics, although they helped my skin, gave me chronic vaginal yeast infections. I just couldn't stand it. I live in a state with a lot of practicing naturopaths, so I decided to give that a try. The visit was very different from the ten-minute dermatology visits I had been used to in the past. The doctor took a very detailed health history, asking questions about the whole of me, not just my face. She emphasized that the goal would be to promote the overall health of my body, not just to suppress the symptoms on my skin. She ordered conventional blood work, but she also ordered tests I had never heard of before that were designed to tell her in detail about the state of my digestive system. I was really glad she did that because I've always had chronic stomach problems, which no doctor had ever really taken seriously.

"Under her direction, I've totally changed my diet. I always knew my way of eating was pretty bad, but I never had anyone encouraging me and supporting me to do it differently. I've eliminated most of the junk food and added food of much higher quality. I'm particularly careful about the types of oil I consume, as I learned, through the naturopath and then firsthand, how much they affected my skin. And I try to remember to take my supplements every day. Not only is my skin much improved, but my energy level has also gone up. As an added bonus, my stomach-aches have almost totally disappeared. I think taking digestive enzymes with every meal and eliminating corn (which we discovered I'm allergic to) did the trick. I have no doubt that all the changes helped my rosacea. I realize now that it was silly to think that rosacea was just something on the outside of me, with no relation to what was going on inside me."

Homeopathy

Homeopathy is a system of medicine that was developed by a German physician named Samuel Hahnemann in the late eighteenth century. The medicine of his time was at best ineffectual and at worst barbaric, and he could not in good conscience continue practicing it. He instead came up with the concept of *similia similibus curentur*, which means "let like be cured by like." Hahnemann wrote: "Every medicine which, among the symptoms it can cause in a healthy body, reproduces those most present in a given disease, is capable of curing the disease in the swiftest, most thorough and most enduring fashion." In other words, homeopathy operates under the principle that any substance that would produce a disease in a healthy person, when given to a sick person with those same disease symptoms, will stimulate a healing response. Although Hahnemann formalized what he called the law of similars in the medical system he called homeopathy, it has actually been mentioned in medical texts as early as the time of Hippocrates.

Homeopathic medicines, called remedies, are minute doses of a wide array of natural substances. Through testing substances on healthy people, called "provings," Hahnemann learned what symptoms a medicine could cause and thus cure. Then through further experimentation, and to his surprise, he found that the more dilute the medicine, the more effective it was.

Homeopathic medicine may sound very strange to those of you who have known only conventional Western medicine, but it was once very popular in this country. In the latter half of the nineteenth century, there were more than twenty homeopathic medical schools. Then, for a number of reasons (including politics and the emergence of antibiotics), it all but disappeared. The rebirth of interest in homeopathy has coincided with the natural health movement in this country. Interestingly, it has always remained a well-utilized form of health care in England, France, Germany, Switzerland, the Netherlands, India, and Latin America.

If you have never seen a homeopath, you are in for a unique experience. The visit is an interview. Since the remedy you are given is based on the totality of symptoms, many of the questions you will be asked will seem to have nothing to do with your rosacea. To a homeopath, the rosacea is just one symptom of the disorder in your being. You are much more than your rosacea, so to find the right medicine, the homeopath will need to ask many questions about your physical, emotional, and mental health.

Chinese Medicine

Chinese medicine is another alternative medical system that may be unfamiliar to you. Diseases are talked about in very non-Western terms, so you may hear expressions like Heat in the Blood with Wind or Heat in the Blood without Wind. You will hear words like Excess and Deficiency, or Yin and Yang. These are all used to describe disharmony in one's body, mind, and spirit.

The Chinese medicine practitioner will ask you many questions about yourself. Your pulse will be taken, but in a very different way than you're used to. There are twenty-eight pulses to be read, and they are an essential part of your diagnosis. It is also common to have your tongue examined; its color, size, and shape will be evaluated and are important to your diagnosis.

Your treatment could consist of acupuncture, Chinese herbs, or both. A well-known Chinese formula indicated for use in rosacea says, "It cools Blood, resolves Dampness, expels Wind and clears Heat from the skin." The language may be foreign to you, but it's a system of medicine that many people use and trust.

Your Own Experimentation: Self-Help Solutions

It's probably a sign of the times, but much of what you'll learn about treatment may come off the Internet, reading about what other people have tried successfully and not so successfully. With rosacea, a lot of what you find out has a hit-or-miss quality to it.

You read about what someone else has discovered, perhaps serendipitously, and you give it a try. You're always hopeful that this will be the "miracle." And then you find that it has a somewhat positive effect, or it has no discernible effect, or, in the worst-case scenario, that it harms your skin. One of the most frustrating things about rosacea (and there are *dozens* of frustrating things) is that there are such differences not only in what aggravates the disorder, but also in what helps it.

Zinc Oxide

One product that most people seem to do well with is zinc oxide. It appears to have an anti-inflammatory action that both decreases redness and reduces the papules and pustules. However, it can be formulated with other ingredients that may cause a negative reaction, so if one brand doesn't work, read the label and try another. Many of you will remember zinc oxide from the days before chemical sunscreens came on the market. Remember those people on the beach with white cream on their noses? The appearance of the regular zinc oxide is an obvious drawback, but there are now clear and flesh-tinted versions on the market. The usual cautionary note is required: Every formulation is different. For example, a product geared toward acne treatment may contain sulfur, and this can adversely affect some rosaceans. It's imperative to always check out the ingredients.

One new product that has gotten good reviews is ZincO, made by Linda Sy Skin Care. Although this product is designed specifically for rosacea, it won't work for everyone, but if it works for you it will perform three or four useful functions. Not only is its anti-inflammatory action healing to the skin, but its flesh-colored tint acts as a concealer. Because of the zinc oxide base, it is a great sunblock that protects your skin from both UVB and UVA rays. It also moisturizes the skin (although those with very dry and sensitive skin will need to apply an additional moisturizer under it to keep the ZincO from flaking). Although the product comes out of the tube with a darkish tint, it has an uncanny ability to blend into even the lightest skin.

Many people who prefer the less expensive plain zinc oxide, but don't want to go around in white face, just use the product at night before bed. People like the benefits of zinc oxide so much that they use a wide variety of products that contain it, ranging from baby diaper cream to calamine lotion.

Julie, who is twenty-five, has not only rosacea, but also seborrheic dermatitis. Her favorite product contains zinc oxide among its ingredients. "I use Rosacea-Ltd III. It is especially formulated for my combination of difficulties—the red face, the flaky skin, and the bumps. It's tinted so I like the way it looks on my skin. But more importantly, my skin likes it."

Other Topical Treatments

Here's something else you might want to try: Some people have achieved excellent results by putting small drops of emu oil, hemp oil, or jojoba oil on their faces. These types of oils seem to do best when applied to a wet face. Not only is the effect anti-inflammatory, but it provides a needed moisturizer for the dry skin that is often a symptom of rosacea (some people have dry skin, others with rosacea have oily skin). George, age forty-nine, swears by a product called A/R Crème that contains emu oil. "It's been great. It also contains zinc oxide and sulfur, which both work for me." As with all rosacea products, some people love it and some don't.

Other rosacea sufferers claim that chamomile soothes their flare-ups. This isn't surprising, since topical chamomile has been shown to have an anti-inflammatory action. One man swears by an herbal cleansing bar with ground chamomile. A woman we know of makes an infusion with chamomile flowers, pouring boiling water on it and then steeping it. When it is no longer hot, she dips in her washcloth and places it on her face. This treatment very successfully eliminates any inflammation she may have.

Another treatment that some people swear by (although it horrifies others) is a vinegar compress. A tablespoon of vinegar is mixed with a pint of lukewarm water. A washcloth soaked in the mixture is placed on the face for fifteen to twenty minutes. Users say rosacea flares can often be eliminated this way.

Nathan, who has had rosacea for the last six years, has his own favorite treatment. "When my face burns and is swollen, I put pure aloe vera all over it. I keep the gel in the refrigerator. The coolness feels so wonderful, and the aloe vera calms down the redness."

Although alpha hydroxy products, because they can irritate the skin, are definitely not for those with rosacea, beta hydroxy products may be very helpful for some. Salicylic acid, the most common of the beta hydroxy acids, is an anti-inflammatory that calms down the skin and removes the flakiness commonly associated with rosacea. This dual-purpose treatment both improves the appearance of the skin and decreases the clogging of the pores. Look for products that contain 1 to 2 percent salicylic acid. Again, as with everything else, the base that the active ingredient is in is vital in preventing a reaction. With this product, a non–water-based version often penetrates the skin most effectively.

Nutritional Solutions

A good nutritional program can diminish the symptoms of rosacea dramatically. This will be addressed in detail in the nutrition chapters in this book.

Taking Care of Your Eyes

Although the more serious eye symptoms associated with rosacea may cause you to consider oral antibiotics and antibiotic ointments, some minor symptoms might respond to non-drug treatments. Dry eyes and blepharitis (inflammation of the eyelid margins), common symptoms of rosacea, seem to respond particularly well to borage and flaxseed oil taken internally. Blepharitis should also be treated with warm washcloth compresses and gentle scrubs of the lid margins. An alternative to the washcloth method is to heat water (not too hot) in a cup in the microwave, dip cottonballs into it, and apply them to closed lids. Repeat several times, reheating the water as necessary.

To scrub the lid, apply diluted baby shampoo or a product made specifically for this purpose to a clean washcloth, and very gently scrub downward. Make sure you're just not cleaning the eyelid skin—instead, concentrate on the lid margins and base of the eyelashes.

After warm compresses and the scrub, consider a lid massage to keep the meibomian glands unplugged. (Remember, these are the glands that, when blocked, cause internal sties and chalazia.) There are different techniques that you can use. One method is to gently make small circles close to the base of your top and bottom eyelid. Another is to take your finger and, lengthwise, roll it from the top of your eyelid down to the eyelashes, and then up toward your eyelashes for the bottom lid. A third technique is to look upward, placing the tip of your finger on a spot near the corner of your lower lid, just under the eyelashes.

Press firmly against the eyeball for a few seconds. Then move your finger along the lid margin to a new area and press again. It should take about five tries to get across the eye. When you're done, repeat the process on your top lid, still looking upward. For all the methods, repeat the motion several times.

Most people with rosacea don't have major ocular problems, but many do find that their eyes feel irritated. A burning sensation is the most common symptom. Because there is decreased tear production, you may want to try eyedrops designed to replenish moisture in dry eyes. There are also ointments designed for the same purpose, but they are best used at bedtime since vision is affected. Unfortunately, the benefits of these products are temporary. Jason, a researcher who spends many hours a week staring at a computer screen, has found a different solution that works for him. "The burning and dryness in my eyes had me wanting to keep them shut most of the day. Obviously, for someone who depends on the computer, that wasn't possible. Then two things happened that have given me tremendous relief. In fact, some days I realize I've gone through the day without once thinking about my eyes. First, I started taking one borage oil capsule, twice a day. The change didn't happen immediately for me, but within a month my eyes felt so much more comfortable. Second, I discovered MSM eyedrops. I'm not exactly sure how they work, but the redness in my eyes has decreased, and my eyes feel normal again." MSM is a biologically available form of sulfur that is a natural product, found in most green plant food and certain algae. It is claimed that the drops, by softening the optical membranes, allow nutrients to pass through to nourish and heal the tissues of the eye. It is worth trying. Not only is it inexpensive, but, more importantly, it may give you relief if you suffer from minor, but unpleasant ocular rosacea symptoms.

There are other simple things to consider that may ameliorate dry, burning eyes. Susan, age fifty-six, says, "My eyes burned all the time. It's an awful feeling. Finally I saw an ophthalmologist who really helped me. He asked me if I was taking any medications and I learned that a whole host of different drugs can cause dry eyes. I finally realized that the medicine I was taking for anxiety was contributing to my problem. The medication was changed and my eyes began to improve. To further help eliminate dry eyes, I use a humidifier when the indoor heating is on, and I make sure that when I use a hair dryer, I keep the airflow away from my eyes. I also avoid smokers like the plague, and I wear glasses in the wind. All these changes have given me a lot of relief."

One cautionary note for those of you who wear eye makeup: Replace it often. If you have any bacterial infection, you don't want to keep re-infecting yourself by using contaminated makeup.

Coping with Flushing and Swelling

Flushing is much more a problem for some people than others, but it can be terribly embarrassing for those who have to deal with it constantly. It gets really old having to tell people, "No, I'm not sunburned." And it's annoying and uncomfortable to deal with the intimation that maybe you're drinking a little too much.

You already know that you have to keep cool (try a nice, refreshing compress), and that you need to drink lots of cold water. If you are self-conscious about your red face, you might want to try two baby aspirin a day, one in the morning and one at night. If you notice bruising or any gastric distress, cut back to only one aspirin a day. (You shouldn't take aspirin at all if you are taking a blood thinner or have a bleeding problem.) An antihistamine a day can also be useful in decreasing your flushing.

The increased blood flow to your face, which gives it that characteristic "rosacea glow," may lead to edema (swelling), which can range from mild to painfully uncomfortable. Just do all the things you know to control flushing—see chapter 4 for tips on controlling your triggers—and the swelling should also improve.

An Abundance of Choices

When it comes to treating your rosacea, you can follow the standard medical route or choose an alternative approach. Or, like more and more Americans, you could decide to combine them, thinking of your choice in treatments like the old Chinese restaurant menus, where you picked one from column A, two from column B, and so on and so on. You may also make the choice to not view rosacea as a separate entity to be treated as such, but instead as a wake-up call to improve the overall health of your body. The point is that you have choices, lots of them—and that's very good news for you. It may take a while to find the right combination, but eventually you'll find it, and you *will* improve. Take your time and try only one innovation at a time, whether it's topical, internal, or behavioral. Otherwise you'll go around in circles trying to figure out what's helping your rosacea and what's aggravating it.

Experiment with different approaches to see what is most helpful for you.

4

Discover Your Triggers—and Learn to Work Around Them

What makes rosacea so frustrating to deal with is that almost any food, drink, activity, or facial product can affect you adversely and trigger a flare-up. It can be amazingly individual; in fact, sometimes, it seems that every person with rosacea has his or her own particular triggers, and what affects one person may not necessarily affect another. Some triggers are virtually universal; others you will have to scout out for yourself. The key to managing rosacea seems to be to keep your face from flushing. You'll definitely need to do some detective work. While there's a wide range of possible triggers, try not to panic—chances are that you're only reactive to some of them. Obviously, you will need to pay close attention for a while to get a sense of what seems to cause flares for you.

Food and Drink

Reactions to food and drink are what most people notice first. Alcoholic beverages are a common trigger, but like all the triggers, this one isn't universal. Some people notice that every type of alcoholic drink affects them, while others have noted that they react only to certain types. Claire, who lives among the many wineries in Sonoma County in northern California, notices that she reacts almost immediately to red wine. White wine doesn't seem to affect her at all, but since she doesn't like white wine, it's not much of a consolation.

Other types of drinks that may affect you are hot liquids, such as tea and coffee. Since the culprit appears to be the heat, not the coffee or tea itself, the key here is to let the drink cool off before you drink it. Make it a habit to wait a few minutes before you take your first sip. If it still seems hot, wait a little longer. Alan has his own little trick. "I get tired of waiting for my coffee to cool off, so I ask for ice water and drop one ice cube into my cup. It speeds everything along, and I can drink along with my companions." You should get used to drinking things warm, instead of hot. The other alternative is to switch to iced versions of your favorite hot drinks.

Many foods, especially spicy ones, can trigger flare-ups. You may not want to hear this, but your days of hot salsa are pretty much over. The chart below will give you an idea of the variety of foods that can cause a reaction.

Common Food Triggers

You will not react to all of these, but you may react to some of them.

BEVERAGES:

✳ Any type of alcohol

✳ Any hot drink

FOODS:

✳ Spicy food, especially hot chiles and pepper

✳ Tomatoes

✳ Chocolate

✳ Citrus fruit

✳ Marinades (depending on ingredients)

✳ Smoked foods

🌺 Vinegar

🌺 Soy sauce

🌺 Hot soups

🌺 Cheese, and possibly other dairy products such as yogurt

🌺 Liver

🌺 Avocados

🌺 Canned tuna

🌺 Bananas

🌺 Lima beans, navy beans, and peas

Histamine-containing foods, or foods that cause a histamine release, can induce flushing. Foods in this category include tomatoes, yogurt, cheese, chocolate, bananas, citrus, canned tuna, avocado, and vinegar. To prevent a reaction to foods high in histamine, it may be beneficial to take an antihistamine two hours before a meal containing such foods. However, since you often don't know what you're going to eat two hours in advance, this can be tricky.

Foods high in niacin, such as liver and yeast, may also cause flushing. Although taking aspirin before a meal may be helpful, you're obviously, not going to consume aspirin every time you eat, so you'll still want to modify your intake of these foods if they cause you to flush. See chapter 7 for information on supplemental niacin that won't cause flushing.

The range of food and drink triggers can make some sufferers experience a kind of "boy in the bubble" syndrome. Ed recalls the weariness and humiliation of declining all the foods and beverages that seem to exacerbate his rosacea. "It can really be a drag," he says, "to inform a hostess that I have to avoid all spices and tomatoes, and to please hold the chocolate sauce on the ice cream. And of course, no wine with dinner. It's not much fun to go to a dinner party and eat the equivalent of oatmeal for the main course and a slice of pound cake for dessert." He says he has learned the advantages of substitution. "It works best if I focus on the things I *can* have," he says, "and there are many of those. The only alternatives are to focus on the negative, or eat and drink things I shouldn't and pay the price. With time, you find the substitutions that fill out the possible menu, and then you don't notice the 'cannots' so much."

Stress

Stress is way up there on the list of triggers. This is truly unfortunate, because it's almost impossible to avoid stress in our daily lives. And yet, if you don't learn to manage stress effectively, combating your rosacea will be far more difficult. Stress can be reduced by exercise, eating properly to regulate your blood sugar, and getting enough sleep.

Conscious stress-management techniques are another vital tool; the method you choose is up to you. Deep breathing will suffice for some people. Dawn, a travel agent, makes a point of practicing this technique at least three times a day. Sitting quietly, she takes twenty deep, rhythmic breaths while visualizing walking by the ocean. "Through years of practice, I've gotten so good at this," she says, "that I can relax almost immediately. Try working all day with the airlines, and you'll get what an accomplishment this is. I used to flush on and off all day. No more, thank goodness." What activity do you find most relaxing? Maybe it's spending time stroking your cat. Or perhaps yoga is your ideal. Make this pursuit a priority in your life—it's absolutely crucial to controlling your rosacea. Please refer to chapter 5 on stress management for additional advice on coping with stress.

Weather

As the saying goes, everyone complains about the weather, but no one does anything about it. That's unfortunate, because the weather can definitely affect rosacea. People vary as far as what bothers them most: the heat, the cold, going from outside where it's hot to inside where it may be air conditioned, or going from the cold outside to the warmth of a heated house. The sun itself, no matter the outside temperature, will often aggravate rosacea. And of course, a cold, brisk wind can bring a flush to just about anyone's face.

Luckily, there are things that you can do to shield your skin from the elements. There are many good reasons to protect yourself from the sun (aside from reducing the risk of skin cancer).

Sun exposure may cause you to overheat, and it can damage the connective tissue in your face, resulting in lymphatic damage. This causes your face to be chronically inflamed, which means it is red all the time. The damage to your connective tissue may also affect your capillaries, making them more fragile and more visible. That's why you must wear a sunscreen or sunblock year round.

Although both protect the skin from both UVA and UVB rays, sunscreens, which contain chemical ingredients, work by absorbing the rays, while blocks work by deflecting them. Sunblock (zinc oxide and titanium dioxide) are easier on the sensitive skin of those with rosacea, and zinc oxide is even beneficial. Never go outside without this protection. Also, get in the habit of wearing a hat that will protect your face from the sun. And of course, even though you wear protection, you should minimize your exposure to the sun, whenever possible. Here's another piece of useful information: New research indicates that supplementing your diet with both mixed carotenoids and Vitamin E (potent antioxidants) offers a protective effect against ultraviolet light (Stahl et al. 2000). The study set out to find out if the oral supplementation would help reduce erythema (redness) after sun exposure. The results showed that the degree of damage to the skin was significantly diminished.

If you find yourself in a situation where it is hot and you are overheating and flushing, suck on ice chips, drink cold drinks, and splash your face with cool water. Jenny and her husband, Stan, both have rosacea. Jenny has had it for years, and Stan just developed it. (No, it's not contagious, just a coincidence.) Jenny is severely reactive to the heat, tending to flush rather dramatically. "I do absolutely everything I can to say cool and avoid flushing. I walk around with those small hand-held fans; I especially like the ones that also spritz cold water on your face." Her husband adds, "Although I don't flare as badly as Jenny does from the heat, we both make sure to drink lots of very cold water, at least eight glasses a day. It really makes a difference for us."

James, who lives in Las Vegas, has his own way of dealing with the heat to prevent flushing. "In the summer, the heat here is unbearable. I'm in and out of my car a lot, so I keep an ice chest in there, loaded with water bottles and washcloths that I've soaked in cold water. When I get in the car, I pat my face and neck with a cloth and drink plenty of ice water. If I am out of my car and feel I'm starting to flush, I'll go into a restroom, dip a paper towel in cold water, and lay it on my face until I cool off. All this has made a huge difference for me."

Cold weather also requires you to protect your skin. Wearing a moisturizer can be very helpful. If it's a particularly windy day, a ski mask will protect you from windburn. At first you may feel awkward in such attire. Anne, a kindergarten teacher, feels like a cat burglar when she walks around her Los Angeles neighborhood with a ski mask covering everything but her eyes. "I try my best not to look suspicious," she jokes. "The school board wouldn't like it if I got arrested for breaking and entering." She adds, "You just have to have a sense of humor about all this. Anyway, I really don't care anymore if I look a little peculiar with my choice of face covering. I just want to protect my skin."

Some people who are really affected by the weather make dramatic changes in their lives. Paula, from Scottsdale, Arizona, went further than most. "I talked to my husband about it at great length," she says, "and he was wonderfully understanding about it. We finally decided that a hot, windy, desert climate was just not compatible with my condition. I was broken out and florid most of the year. We moved to San Diego, arranging a transfer within our current company, and my face looked better almost immediately. We actually wound up liking it better anyway." Paula's sister, also a rosacea sufferer, lives in Minnesota, and finds the cold weather there disturbs her skin almost as much as the sun in Arizona tormented her sister. She is planning a move to California when her son graduates from high school.

Of course, not everyone has the ability or opportunity to just pick up and move to a more accommodating climate. But if you can and you have an adventurous spirit, consider it as an option if you live in a part of the country that is really hard on your skin.

Exercise

There is no doubt that exercise causes flushing, and yet there is also no doubt that exercise is vital to your physical and emotional well-being. Don't use your rosacea as an excuse to be a coach potato. Sure, you have rosacea, but the vast majority of people with this condition are not sick, weak, or limited in any way. It's important that you remember that, and maintain a regular exercise program for optimal health and stress reduction.

All you have to do is modify your workout patterns. If you exercise inside, get a fan and keep cool water and ice chips close at hand. If you exercise outside, wear your sunblock and hat, and venture outdoors in the early morning or in the early evening. Bring cool water with you to drink or to splash on your face if necessary. You can also put cold water in a spray bottle and spray yourself when you feel you are overheating. There are body-cooling neck wraps that you can buy that will actually lower your body temperature by cooling the carotid arteries. This creates a cooling system for the whole body and gives you another tool to avoid overheating.

George, a bank executive who has had rosacea for nine years, likes to run on an outdoor track at sunset. Not only does he not have to deal with the sun shining down on him, but he loves the serenity of that time of day, plus the fact that he often has the track all to himself. "I can't understand why for years I ran in full sunlight," he says. "I always got overheated and noticed a definite increase in redness. Running in the evening is by far more enjoyable. I feel great when I'm done, and it's a good substitute for the evening cocktail I used to drink, which is something else that doesn't work too well with rosacea and me." George has the right idea. He knew that exercise was something that should never be eliminated. He actually exercises more now, because he discovered that his energy level increased when the sun wasn't beating down on him. The resultant sense of well-being from taking care of his body has made the elimination of alcohol from his life much easier. He acknowledges that he is actually grateful that the rosacea gave him the impetus to no longer have drinking be an important part of his life.

Skin-Care Products

When you have rosacea, it seems like you're constantly doing something to your face. There's always some new product that you think might be helpful. The problem is that most people with rosacea have hyperirritable skin that can't tolerate certain creams, cosmetics, and ointments. In many ways, it becomes a system of trial and error. You just don't know ahead of time how you will respond. Wanda learned this firsthand. "I was giving an important presentation to a conference of my peers. I wanted everything to be perfect. The night before the presentation, I noticed some blotches on my skin and decided to use a cream that other rosacea sufferers had raved about. The next morning my face was completely inflamed. I was just mortified. I gave my speech that day, feeling totally self-conscious. But I learned an important lesson that I've never forgotten. Now when I try a new product, I choose days when I know I don't need to see anyone or do any business. Then, if my face flares, I can deal with it, without adding any undue stress to the situation."

There are certain products that you should definitely avoid. The most common irritant is anything with alcohol in it. Also be wary of any skin-care products containing witch hazel, peppermint, eucalyptus oil, or menthol. Make sure to avoid products with alpha hydroxy acids. Fragrances in skin products can be a problem as well. If you use hair spray, do not let it touch your face. Use one hand as a shield as you spray with the other. It took Joyce, a college student, almost a year to figure out that hair spray was causing her face to flare. "I was mystified as to what was irritating my skin. I had actually eliminated all face products except for a gentle cleanser (which I kept changing in frustration), and yet kept thinking I was missing something. One day, it finally occurred to me that my hair spray actually ended up misting onto my face. I just never thought of it being a problem, because it wasn't something I was applying directly to my skin. I stopped using it, and almost immediately my complexion improved."

You will discover firsthand the other ingredients that you personally will need to avoid. An instant clue is something that stings or burns. Rinse your face with cold water immediately, and keep rinsing until the offending product is completely removed and your face no longer burns. Also make sure that the products you use don't clog your pores, by buying only those labeled as noncomedogenic. Because you'll have to throw out much of what you buy, it's wise to purchase the smallest sizes you can. Sample sizes are best if you can get them. More and more companies that sell products for people with sensitive skin are selling small amounts for you to try. It's worth it to them, because it gets you to try their product. The benefit to you is that if it irritates your face, which unfortunately is often the case, you're not out much money. Another option is to try to buy from a store that allows returns. Regardless, don't be afraid to ask for your money back if you're truly dissatisfied with a product. You may not get a refund, but it's worth a try.

One further wrinkle to deal with and prepare yourself for: You will find a product that your skin seems to thrive on, and then one day it won't. Just like that. One woman we talked to compared it to feeding a cat. "You work so hard finding something they'll eat, and then you think you have it. You get so excited that you buy cans and cans of something like Gourmet Feast or some other supposedly tasty treat. And as soon as you do that, they go off it and won't touch it. It's like they decided overnight that you were trying to poison them. That's how I see my skin sometimes. It's as crazy as my cat."

Cleaning Your Face

Let's assume that you have found a gentle, nonabrasive cleanser that you like. There are many cleansers on the market, so if one doesn't work, simply try another. Some companies make both bar and liquid versions of the same product; you may find that the bar form is fine and the liquid irritating, or vice versa. This is because the two forms may have different ingredients. It's important to pay close attention to labels, just as you do for the foods you purchase.

Now that you've chosen a product, it's important to keep your face clean, but in a way that causes no irritation to the skin. Spread the cleanser gently on your face with your fingertips. Do not use a washcloth. Rinse with plenty of lukewarm water. Finally, blot your face dry with a soft towel. It's important not to rub it dry. Better yet, if possible, let your skin air dry. Then wait a while before applying anything to your face. Some people need to wait as long as thirty minutes, others only five. The important thing is to wait until you can apply moisturizers or other products without feeling a stinging sensation. Increase the waiting time as needed. If the stinging continues, discard the product. This cleansing process should be done twice a day.

Shaving

In addition to cleansing their faces, most men must go through the ordeal of shaving. You may find that an electric shaver is less irritating to your skin. If, however, you need the closeness of a blade, make sure that it's sharp, and think about shaving in the shower. The added moisture will enable you to come through your shave with much less irritation. If you want to use an aftershave, make sure it is alcohol-free. If you can't find one in your local pharmacy, explore the shelves of stores that carry more natural products.

Bathing

Both showering and bathing can bring on the flush. That's how Ron, a psychologist, discovered his first trigger. "I'd wake up in the morning, and staring at my face in the mirror while brushing my teeth, I looked like a normal fifty-year-old man. Then I'd take my shower. I always like them really hot, probably from growing up in the cold winters of Connecticut. I'd get out of the shower, and my face looked like it had been baked in the oven for forty-five minutes. I'd then spend the morning with a lobster-red face. Everyone would want to know how I managed to get so sunburned in the middle of the winter. Actually, one of my clients told me what was going on. He was more knowledgeable about rosacea than I. Needless to say, my days of hot showers are over."

But of course, you can't forgo your daily ablutions. Keep in mind that showering is better than taking a bath, because you can make heat adjustments more easily. Shorten the time of your shower, and instead of hot water, lower the temperature to lukewarm. You can also take a California drought shower, which means shutting the water off while you're soaping up your body and hair. Another trick is to suck on ice chips while showering. (A tip from one woman, who does this routinely, is to use a plastic glass or cup for safety's sake.)

If your face is still aggravated after your shower, there are a couple of other things to consider. Remember that your shampoo and conditioner may come into direct contact with your face, and you might be reacting to them. If that's the case, it would be a good idea to try more natural products. And lastly, as strange as it seems, some people are so sensitive that they even react to the chlorine in the water. If that's the case, think about installing a water filter in your shower. All these modifications will enable you to leave the shower with a minimum of flushing. You'll be pleasantly surprised at how well these few tricks work, and you'll no longer dread the side effects of keeping yourself clean.

Sex

This is one trigger that you won't hear about from your dermatologist or read about in the little handouts they give you. It's something you figure out yourself if you have rosacea. It only makes sense doesn't it? Sex, if you're doing it right, is going to make you flush. It's got it all—the heat, the exertion, the hormonal stimulation. Just the rubbing alone of an unshaven man's cheek against a woman's can cause considerable irritation if her skin is hypersensitive.

It's embarrassing to have everyone know when you've just finished making love. But your flushed face may be a dead give-away to people who know you well.

So, make sure that your bedroom has a good fan, and, if you're in a climate that gets really hot, use air-conditioning. A spray bottle of cold water is another a good idea. And of course, keep an ice-cold drink of water near your bed. If you stay cooled down, your private life will remain just that—private.

Drug-Induced Flare-ups

Certain medications used in the treatment of cardiovascular diseases, called vasodilators, cause flushing and subsequent aggravation of rosacea. If you are on such medication, discuss the issue with your physician and try to find an alternative treatment.

Topical steroids prescribed for rosacea can also cause considerable problems. Initially, these drugs seem to help with inflammation. But ultimately, they will only make existing rosacea worse. In fact, they can actually cause rosacea-like symptoms in people who are using them on their faces for some other condition. Remember, it isn't worth the short-term amelioration of symptoms to do this damage to your skin.

Triggers That May Surprise You

As you may already know, or are getting closer to realizing, this is one strange disorder you have. The one common denominator to avoid at all costs is flushing, although some people have very little and others of us could lead Santa's sleigh. (You've just got to laugh about it sometimes!) You will discover your personal triggers and create ways of dealing with them that are totally unique to you. For example, an unusual trigger that some people have been noting is fluorescent lighting; it causes them to flare. You can try to avoid places with this type of lighting— unfortunately a difficult task in this day and age—or you can go bravely forth and do what you need to do to protect your face. One woman we know of uses an umbrella indoors when in this situation. Others would prefer to just flare.

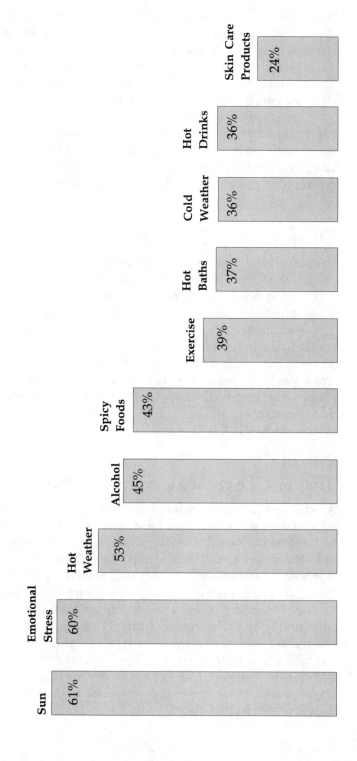

Chart From the National Rosacea
Society: Most Common Rosacea Tripwires

Sun 61%
Emotional Stress 60%
Hot Weather 53%
Alcohol 45%
Spicy Foods 43%
Exercise 39%
Hot Baths 37%
Cold Weather 36%
Hot Drinks 36%
Skin Care Products 24%

Jennifer, an accountant, had to quit her aromatherapy sessions. Though nothing was put directly on her face, the volatile oils that are used become vapor, and the fine particles floating in the air landed on her face, causing it to burn. "I can't even be around someone wearing lavender oil, which is not that rare an occurrence in northern California," she says.

Paying close attention to even the smallest things can yield valuable information. Henry, a college instructor, noticed that most of the problems on his face occurred on the right side. "It took me about five years to figure it out. I sleep on my stomach with my right cheek against the pillow. I don't know if it was something on the pillow, maybe an allergen, or detergent, or just the pressure of my face being pressed against the pillow, but when I switched to sleeping on my back, the appearance of my face definitely improved."

If you are convinced you have a trigger that you've never read or heard about, trust yourself and believe that it's real. It may not be the norm, but then again, what about rosacea is? On the previous page is a chart of the most common triggers.

Below you'll find a checklist that can help you determine your triggers. Make copies of it and fill one out every day until you feel that you have a handle on what tends to aggravate your rosacea. This may take weeks, since multiple triggers can confuse the picture. If, for example, you're not sure which of two foods is causing a flare, don't eat them together for a while. Let's say that you think that you're reacting to chocolate and tomatoes. Don't have a meal of spaghetti and then chocolate cake for dessert. If you end up with a bumpy or flushed face, you'll have no idea what caused it. Eat the spaghetti with tomato sauce by itself. Then wait and watch for a couple of days. Then do the same with a piece of chocolate. Doing it this way, you have a better idea of which foods are fine and which you need to be cautious about. When you feel you have identified a trigger, eliminate it and see what happens.

Do the same thing with anything you actually put on or near your face. You'll have to distinguish between face creams, suncreens and blocks, cleansers, makeup, and more. The important thing is to be patient. Go slow and pay careful attention—and rest assured that you'll soon understand how to keep your own particular case of rosacea under control.

Rosacea Diary Checklist

Use this form at the end of each day to identify your personal rosacea tripwires.

Date:

Check the weather conditions you were exposed to today.

☐ Sun   ☐ Heat   ☐ Cold   ☐ Humidity   ☐ Wind

Check the foods, beverages and other items you ingested today.

☐ Spicy foods   List: _____

☐ Alcohol   List: _____

☐ Hot beverages   List: _____

☐ Fruits   List: _____

☐ Dairy products   List: _____

☐ Vegetables   List: _____

☐ Drugs   List: _____

☐ Other   List: _____

Check the conditions and activities you experienced today.

☐ Emotional stress   Describe: _____

☐ Physical exertion   Describe: _____

☐ Hot bath/sauna

☐ Warm room temperatures

☐ Medical condition   List: _____
            (flushing, chronic cough, hot flashes, fever, etc.)

☐ Other   List: _____

Check the substances you came in contact with today.

☐ Skin care products   List: _____

☐ Cosmetics   List: _____

☐ Soap   List: _____

☐ Perfume   List: _____

☐ Aftershave   List: _____

☐ Shampoo   List: _____

☐ Household products   List: _____

☐ Other   List: _____

What is the condition of your rosacea today?

☐ No flare-up   ☐ Mild flare-up   ☐ Severe flare-up

Did you comply with your medical therapy today?
☐ Yes   ☐ No

Chart courtesy of National Rosacea Society

5

Stress Management

For many people, stress is the number-one trigger for rosacea flare-ups. It's also a very complicated subject in its own right. As you can imagine, these two conditions intersect in some complex ways. It's not enough that daily life presents much to be stressed about, but rosacea itself, with its wide array of symptoms and necessary lifestyle changes, can be the biggest stress inducer of all. For your emotional sanity, and for the sake of your face, you have to learn to control the stress in your life.

How Do I Know If I'm Stressed?

There are many tests, some of them complex, that can help you gauge your levels of both mental stress and physical stress. But there are also simple indicators of which you should be aware. Here are some for you to consider:

Mental/Emotional Stress

❊ Feelings of depression

❊ Feelings of anxiety

❊ Confusion

❊ Irritability

❋ Agitation

❋ Loss of interest in sex, food, or life in general

❋ Sudden abuse of drugs, alcohol, or cigarettes

❋ Frequent negative thoughts

❋ Nightmares

❋ Inability to concentrate

❋ Hyperactivity or listlessness

❋ Nervousness

❋ Feelings of worthlessness or low self-esteem

Physical Stress

❋ Sleeplessness

❋ Headaches

❋ Dizziness

❋ Upset stomach

❋ Frequent need to use the bathroom

❋ Loose stools or constipation

❋ Light-headedness

❋ Involuntary clenching of jaws or fists

❋ Tightness in any muscle group

❋ Higher-than-normal blood pressure

❋ Racing heart or irregular heartbeat

❋ Sweatiness or clammy feelings in any body part

❋ Lack of energy

❋ Change in appetite

There is a very simple test, if you live in the Western world, to determine whether or not you are stressed. Here it is: Get a small feather (your down comforter is a great source). Close your mouth and hold the feather under your nostrils. Breathe. If the feather moves, you have stress!

Who Do You Think You Are?

Isn't it strange that the most misleading statements frequently begin with the phrase "I AM . . ."? There is no verb, in any language, more important than the verb "to be," yet no verb is more often abused. "I AM" is inevitably followed by a string of words that very definitely do *not* define who you are.

As a little infant, you act as if "I AM a mouth." Everything—mother's nipple, my big toe, my sister's pencil—gets fused with "me." Later on, having laboriously developed an ego, you believe that your identity is your name, e.g., "I AM Larry." After your range of social contacts has been widened a bit, you begin to identify with the notion of relationships, e.g., "I AM Isaac's son." Later still, you believe that your job defines who you are, e.g., "I AM a businessman." In between, you begin to identify with attributes, emotions, and mental states, e.g., "I AM thin" or "I AM angry" or "I AM confused." Attributes are particularly dangerous if you identify with a symptom, a disease, or the idea of being a helpless victim, e.g., "I AM nauseous" or "I AM a diabetic" or "I AM an incest survivor."

This is the trap of experiencing any illness, including rosacea. If you speak of yourself as "I AM a rosacea sufferer," then that tag becomes a significant part of your identity and your future.

The most pervasive misidentification of all, however, comes from your "personal myth" or "personal story." Meet somebody for the first time, win her confidence, and extend the invitation: "I've an hour to spare just now, and would love to get to know you." She will string together a bunch of memories that may or may not be representative of the billions of experiences she's actually had. These form her identity, self-perception, or personal myth.

Depending on whether or not this myth is essentially of violence, of love, of success, of failure, of victimhood, of illness, or of health, you can be pretty sure that this identity will follow her into her future and determine her happiness level.

Nobody, it seems, deals adequately with any mishap, illness, or vicissitude of life without tweaking or substantially revising their personal myth or personal worldview. Recovery from any difficult circumstance, including illness, is closely tied to reperceiving and redefining your own story. And this redefining makes it easier to change your behavior in the future. No change can be sustained without behavioral modification, and no major change can be sustained without significant and sustained behavioral modification.

Dealing with stress, then, as a first step means wrestling with an adequate answer to the question "Who am I?" Hinduism has a wonderful saying, "I have a body, but I am not my body; I have emotions, but I am not my emotions; I have an intellect, but I am not my intellect; I have a personality, but I am not my personality." When you think about it, it's foolish to believe that you are your physical body. For example, you shed fifty million body cells per minute. You slough off 95 percent of your body's cells in less than a year, and simply manufacture new lookalikes from your food and drink, from the air you breathe, and from the sunlight that gets reflected onto your retinas.

Chances are that you do much of your grocery shopping at the same store. Next time you're there, notice the people wheeling out carts laden with goodies. And yet the store never appears to be depleted. Each time you go to the store, you know exactly in which aisle to get your milk, your bananas, and your bread. It's as if as the clerk passes your carton of eggs across the beeping glass plate, some microchip-entity monk under the counter says, "One dozen organic, free range, jumbo-sized, fertile, brown eggs. Please replace!" And a dutiful gnome dashes out from the storeroom and obliges. It's as if the store isn't so much a physical building full of physical produce as it is a software program full of intelligence. Your body is somewhat like that—some extraordinary intelligence is organizing the shedding and the acquiring of old cells and new cells, according to some unique blueprint that defines you.

Buttercups and caterpillars both take in the same basic building blocks of matter (carbon, hydrogen, oxygen, and nitrogen molecules) from nutrients in the soil, air, and sunlight and build them into buttercups and caterpillars. They never get it wrong. Have you ever seen a "catercup" or a "butterpillar"? Moreover, you and your friend, though both of you manage to build humans of these materials, always succeed in following your own totally unique blueprints. You never confuse your image in the mirror with that of your friend's.

So who are you? Obviously not just your physical body. Don't you feel better already? Who then? The great mystics of all traditions give the same answer: "I AM." Not a mouth, name, relationship, attribute, job, set of memories, or personal myth. And certainly not a skin disease. Just the core essence. Could you hang out for a while in that realization? It'll do wonders for you.

Meditation

For over nine thousand years, the greatest teachers have declared that meditation is the surest way to that kind of dis-identification. Meditation comes in many stripes and several schools, and the ultimate objective of meditation goes far beyond physical, emotional, or mental well-being. But even if you are only interested in these three by-products, you'd be well served by learning to meditate.

For those of you who don't have a meditation practice, here is an extremely simple style called "mantra meditation." Put simply, it means repeating a word or phrase for the duration of the meditation. It can be a sacred word, from any spiritual tradition, or any mundane word of your choice. The idea is to fend off all distractions (physical sensations, ideas, memories, fantasies) by coming back to the mantra as soon as you realize you're off on a tangent. It's not a competition, and there is no need to grade your effort or judge yourself. You'll probably find that the distractions occur several times a minute—no big deal, just go back to the mantra each time you become aware of the sideshow.

Even five minutes a day helps. It's better if you can do two sessions a day, and doing two sessions of fifteen minutes each is preferable to doing one session of thirty minutes. Experiment with three things. First, the time of the day. Depending on your natural biological rhythms, you may find that some times of the day work better than others. At these optimal times, you should be able to experience an alert relaxation. Second, experiment with the location. For some the best place will be outdoors in a quiet spot; for others it will be in a darkened room (with perhaps a candle, incense, or very soft music). Quietness is of the essence. Third, experiment with body posture. You've no doubt seen pictures of cross-eyed yogis in impossible-looking full-lotus positions. But good results are possible in any position—standing, kneeling, sitting, squatting—as long as you maintain a straight spine.

Visualization

For those who find that meditation smacks of the esoteric, how about just using your imagination? Can you imagine a rabbit just now? How about a pink rabbit? Well, how about a pink rabbit with an elf on its back? See, your imagination works perfectly. Why not make it work to reduce your stress level? Here's a simple exercise:

Sit or lie down, and close your eyes. Imagine that you are standing at the side of a large swimming pool, which has a sloping floor. It's filled, not with water, but with a healing energy-light (in your favorite color).

Now begin walking very slowly and intentionally into the shallow end. Feel the healing energy on the soles of your feet; trickling ticklingly between your toes; covering your heels and ankles and insteps; and moving up along your shins and calves. You can feel it not just at skin level, but in the flesh and muscle and bones and ligaments and tendons. Everywhere it touches it soothes. And each time you breathe out now, you can let go of any tension in that part of your body and relax.

You continue walking deeper into the pool, and now you feel the healing energy move through your knees and up through your thighs, up to your buttocks and genitals and abdomen. Once again it heals to the core, bringing peace and tranquility. And each time you breathe out now, you can let go of any tension in that part of your body and relax some more.

You move deeper still. And now the healing energy moves up into your chest and up along your spinal column, touching and soothing all of the internal organs: your heart and lungs and kidneys and liver. And each organ feels serene and in perfect harmony. And each time you breathe out now, you can let go of any tension in that part of your body and relax even more fully.

Deeper yet. Now you feel it in your shoulders, and you realize that your fingers, hands, forearms, biceps, and triceps are all bathing serenely in it. And each time you breathe out now, you can let go of any tension in that part of your body and relax even more deeply.

Finally, you submerge yourself totally in this healing energy-light, and you feel it move up along your throat and neck, into your jaw and mouth, into your cheeks and nostrils, into your eyes and ears; up the sides and back of your head and up your forehead, right up to the crown of your head. And it seeps soothingly into your innermost brain—healing your memories, your thinking, your will, your dreams, your fears. Everything is at peace, everything is tranquil, everything is serene. And each time you breathe out now, you can let go of any tension in that part of your body and relax totally.

As you end the visualization, give yourself the following post-visualization suggestion: "For the rest of the day, whether

I'm at work or at play, with each in-breath I will take in peace, and with each out-breath I will let go of tension and toxicity."

Quality Worry-Time

Perhaps you're a pragmatist and just can't see yourself meditating or visualizing. "Fantasy is for those who want to escape reality," is your belief. Okay, let's get real here. You're stressed, right? You're worried about real stuff, right? You probably catch yourself fretting all through the day, whenever you can afford the luxury of "free time." Well, then here's an exercise tailor-made for you.

A dedicated stess-gourmet like you deserves to be taken seriously, and your stressors need to be honored. It's fine for irresponsible types to dismiss their cares with a silly song like "Don't worry, be happy." But you are a mature citizen. You take your duties seriously. If you don't do the worrying, then who in God's name will? You deserve to be recognized for dedication above and beyond the call of duty, so this next exercise is specially dedicated to you.

Your assignment is to promise the nagging anxiety at your elbow "quality worry-time" on a daily basis, on the understanding that it keep its distance the rest of the time. But you have to keep your part of the bargain. Faithfully, steadfastly, anal-retentively, you must sit down daily for the agreed-upon period of time and record all your worries—meticulously. Worst-case scenarios deserve a preeminent place.

Review this journal regularly. You'll find two things, even after years of scribing. First, you haven't died yet. And second, you very probably have found that the same issues keep raising their heads. Shouldn't these two results tell you something? Like beauty, anxiety is in the "I" of the beholder. In *Hamlet*, Shakespeare made a good point about psychology: "There is nothing either good nor bad, but thinking makes it so."

Get a Hobby

What Shakespeare did for fun, apart from writing sonnets and composing Oscar-winning–type dramas, is really not known. Golf had not yet been invented, and he probably wasn't into stamp collecting. But hobbies are a powerful way of reducing stress. Chances are that if you have rosacea, your face has been your chief hobby. You have probably been more concerned and more creative about its welfare than about most other things in your life. Here's some advice: Give it a break; take it out of the lime-light; promote something else to center stage. The synonym "pas-time" is unfortunate since it gives the impression that a hobby is merely a way of killing those long spaces between more useful and productive activities. The truth is that hobbies, fully embraced, can focus your attention away from your face and onto life-enhancing and stress-reducing activities. They can create for you like-minded communities with common interests, and the opportunity for companionship and good times.

Since it is typically both freely chosen and not concerned about "making a living," a hobby has a very freeing and creative effect on the personality. Since you are really doing it "for the fun of it," it releases all of those happy childhood memories. Nature, in her generosity and wisdom, adds in for good measure endorphins that flood the system with pleasure.

Your hobby, if properly chosen, can tap into a treasure trove of buried ecstasy and biochemical "highs." Play is not just some-thing that kids were meant to do until they grew up, got sense, and took responsibility for life. It is a carefully thought-out evolu-tionary strategy that fuels the thrust toward mental, emotional, and physical well-being.

A hobby, then, is not just about taking your mind off your face, it is about claiming your inheritance as a work of art in prog-ress. You are many times more creative than you have given yourself credit for. Think of all the things that you have wanted to do, to try some day. Get a piece of paper and write them down, then check them out by surfing the Web, talking to friends, visit-ing the library, signing up for classes. Decide what activities appeal to you most and give them a try.

Gimme That Ol' Time Religion

If you have been reading the newspapers lately, you'll certainly have seen that some serious scientific research has been going on in the areas of prayer and religious observance. In the last thirty years, more than 150 carefully devised, controlled, randomized studies of prayer have been carried out; most have shown statisti-cally significant results. The researchers have been creative in devising scientific tests to gauge the effects of prayer on the well-being of enzymes, yeasts, bacteria, viruses, plants, animals, and human beings. In studying humans, these experiments have looked at interventions in both physical and psychological healing. One study by O'Laoire (1997) showed that being prayed for at a distance had a very highly statistical influence on the levels of self-esteem, anxiety, and depression of the subjects being prayed for. A more intriguing finding of this study was that there was an even more significant positive influence on the mental and emotional well-being of those who actually did the praying.

Anxiety, depression, and poor self-esteem are well-proven consequences of out-of-control stress. O'Laoire's study showed that people who perceived themselves to be managing their stress well had lower levels of anxiety and depression and higher levels of self-esteem. Prayer then has the ability to reduce the stresses that trigger rosacea.

Sociologists of religion have accrued an impressive body of demographic information showing very impressive gains to people with a regular religious practice. This may, of course, be a result of several factors: It may be that "religious" people are less likely to indulge in destructive habits like smoking or drinking to excess; or it may be that belonging to a community, at a time when the modern trend is increasingly toward isolated individuality, is itself health promoting; or perhaps the self-transcending effect of a belief in a caring God is very freeing, thus conferring both psychological and physical aftereffects.

Whatever the reason and whatever the mechanism, the scientific data suggests that there is value in prayer and in religious commitment, whatever particular form it takes. If you're so inclined, give it a try.

Quality Time Off

Americans tend to live their work week in a highly paid form of bondage. Never in the history of the planet have people wanted so badly to bargain away health, family, and "free" time for a share in the affluent American dream. Whatever happened to summer holidays? Remember how it felt to be a kid on the last day of school? Think seriously about your job. Is it allowing you enough free time to enjoy your life, or is it just your major source of stress?

Regular "time off" is vital to physical, mental, and emotional well-being. It's an interesting phrase, "time off." What does it suggest? Does it imply that work is what life is really about, and vacation is permission to opt out of this rat race for a brief period? Or does it mean that time is a made-up pressure cooker and every so often we come to our senses and turn it off, so as to see what life is really about? Hopefully, it's the latter.

In practice, what would it look like to really take time for yourself? It should have a daily, weekly, monthly, and annual aspect. Here is an example of a well-rounded schedule: Each day, build into your timetable an hour of fun—a massage, a swim, coffee with a friend. Each week, take a full day off for rest and relaxation—the beach, a hike, golf, a drive in the country. Once a month, take a full weekend off, Friday evening through Sunday evening—a ski trip, a meditation retreat, a seminar on a topic that interests you, a get-together with your co-hobbyists. Then annually, a decent vacation of at least two weeks' length—to travel to some exotic spot; or simply hole up at home with the shades down and the phone, fax, and e-mail unplugged. If your job won't allow you that much time off, you're in the wrong job. If you think about it, overwork may well be the single greatest destroyer of physical health, emotional stability, mental tranquility, and interpersonal relationships.

Get a Companion Animal

One of the things you needed most in life—and probably didn't get—was unconditional love. It was the beginning of your stress. Children have to become very creative to garner the love that is their birthright, but which is often doled out in pitifully inadequate amounts, laced with rules, prohibitions, and the withholding of affection for minor mistakes. Life becomes a game in which you walk the tightrope between being yourself and risking censure, all in an attempt to maximize the love and regard from others that is the core currency of self-esteem.

So you didn't get unconditional love as a kid. And you're not getting a whole lot of it now. What to do? Get a pet! Maybe a pet lizard isn't quite going to do it for you, but a dog will. If you really want to experience the loyalty and commitment of a soul who reads you deeply and loves you anyway, get a canine. Save an older animal from a local shelter, and the love you'll get will be overwhelming. Watch your stress levels plummet as your contentment and joy increase. You have someone who loves you, but better yet, you have someone to love.

There are some people who believe that cats are for those who are interested in giving unconditional love to a soul who couldn't care less. But then they've never had the opportunity to really bond with a cat. They're definitely different from dogs, but they're equally wonderful companion animals. Ask cat lovers how it feels to have a cat curled up next to them, gently purring, and looking up at them with those soft, beautiful eyes. The cat, by its very nature, is a companion with whom to relax and be calm.

Strangely enough, every time we speak, even to human friends, our blood pressure jumps several points. It seems that we are always unconsciously fearful of being judged when we open our mouths. However, when we speak to animals, there is no elevation in blood pressure. Evidently, even in the deep unconscious, we understand animals love us unconditionally.

There is a substantial body of research showing the positive impact of having a pet on many facets of physical and mental health. Petting a cat's head or scratching a dog's belly is not just something you are doing for the animal's pleasure. It's as therapeutic for you as is deep breathing or a letter from a close friend.

Stroke sometimes results in receptive aphasia, which is the inability to understand language. The victim struggles to make sense of even the simplest of spoken sentences. But there is frequently a very interesting and beneficial side effect: The right brain takes up the slack and significantly improves a person's ability to read subtle body language, particularly the facial language of lips, eyebrows, and smile lines. The result is that they can almost unerringly detect untruth and dissembling in others. Perhaps that is something animals give us—their understanding of verbal language may be limited, but they watch intently as we interact with them and read our moods, needs, and affects. An hour with your dog is worth two hours on a psychologist's couch.

The Here and Now

Basically, stress is the experience of being out of alignment with our true nature. Like a shoulder out of its socket, this generates lots of pain and anxiety. Stress was meant to equip us to deal with *real* problems in the *real* here and *real* now. Unfortunately, humans can have have stress reactions over imaginary problems in the future and remembered problems from the past. And we manifest the physical, emotional, and mental symptoms of those future and past issues in the present. Obviously, this is a time-consuming and destructive response.

Try this instead: Think of animals like gazelles in Africa. They only worry about real lions during real hunts in real time. Be a gazelle and live fully in the present.

6

The Coverup—from Makeup to Laser

Disguising Rosacea

If your rosacea is not yet under control, you're definitely not happy with the appearance of your skin. And even if your rosacea is under control, you may not be happy with the appearance of your skin. Over the years, rosacea can take its toll on your face. In other chapters of this book, we talk about dealing with rosacea from the inside out. This chapter is about treating the exterior—making your face look as normal as possible.

The Makeover

In most native cultures, it is the men who wear the makeup, but that's not the case in our modern Western world. This is an area where women have the decided advantage, because most of us have been experimenting with makeup since our early teenage years. It's natural for us to know how to enhance some parts of our face and camouflage others. For men, this is a lot more difficult. Not only do they not have the skill, but they also feel silly and self-conscious walking around wearing makeup. The truth is, however, that if you're a man with rosacea, you too have the right to improve your appearance any way you want. We're not suggesting mascara (unless that's a particular desire of yours), but there's absolutely no reason why you can't use foundation or powders to improve the appearance of your skin. You just need to practice using them so that your face looks as natural as possible. (This is true for women too.) The whole point of properly applied makeup, with or without rosacea, is to look like you're not wearing any. If you're a man and you feel overwhelmed by this, you might ask a woman friend to work with you on learning to apply makeup. Whatever your sex, if you don't know quite what to do, professionals who work with people with skin disorders can show you the best possible technique.

Robert, a thirty-five-year-old businessman, left his old biases behind and now regularly wears makeup to cover his red face. "Originally, I was horrified at the idea," he says. "But I was also horrified at having to deal with clients every day with a face that was often severely flushed. I had the good fortune to end up dating a woman who also had rosacea. One day she was making up her face and insisted on doing the same for me. I refused for weeks, but when my face was really flaring, I gave in. I finally realized it was no big deal. Most days, if I'm under control, I just put on a couple drops of jojoba oil to moisturize my skin and then top that with a tinted zinc oxide. If it's a bad face day, I'll use a foundation and a little powder. I haven't gotten up the nerve to buy cosmetics in a department store yet, but since I can get just about anything I want through mail order these days, that's not a problem. The important thing is that I feel better about my appearance. It's silly to get hung up on the idea that wearing makeup is a 'girl thing.'"

We won't even try to recommend a particular line of cosmetics, since every person with rosacea seems to have their own idiosyncratic response to everything on the planet. However, the best results often come from products that are as natural as possible, with few preservatives. Visit your local health food emporium and try some of their cosmetics, or look on the Internet and see what you can find. Many companies that cater to people with sensitive skin will give refunds if you react adversely to their product.

Another trick to try is green-tinted creams or powders. Apply them lightly and then cover them over with a base. The theory here is that green neutralizes the redness. These products work for some, but others feel they just make their skin look green or muddy brown.

There are those with rosacea who prefer to use no makeup at all. Their instinct is to let their inflamed skin rest as much as possible and not burden it with anything extra. On the other hand, those with more severe rosacea, especially if they're out there in public view, may feel that they have no choice.

Facials

You end up putting so much on your skin that sometimes you really would love for it to have a deep cleaning. And to have it feel pampered, after all it's been through, would be bliss. But facials can be a scary business: To have someone who doesn't know your skin do new and different things to it may make you so tense that you won't be able to enjoy the process at all. And yet, if a facial is done by the right person, you can come through it just fine. The problem is, of course, finding the right person.

Jacy tells this story of trial and error. "I was given a referral from my dermatologist to a local aesthetician who supposedly treats lots of people with rosacea. I noticed during the facial that my face burned a lot, but I figured she knew what she was doing. After all, she was recommended by my doctor. When it was over, she sold me lots of products that would be 'good' for me. When I got into my car, I looked into the mirror for the first time. I had totally flared. My face was red and blotchy—it looked terrible and stayed that way for weeks. I was, of course, afraid to try any of the products she had given me. I threw them all away, because I didn't trust her judgment at all. I was so upset, and I thought the experience meant that I could never have another facial.

"A couple of years later, staring in dismay at my skin and the embedded blackheads that I just couldn't get rid of, I decided to try a facial one more time. In the phone book, I saw an ad for a woman who treated those with sensitive skin and rosacea, and I decided to give her a try. This was a very different experience. Every time she put something on my face, she'd ask how it felt. If there was even the slightest tingling, she'd remove it. She used all natural products, and when she was done, she made sure to put on a vasoconstricting [the opposite of dilating] cream to guard against any redness. I walked out of there very slightly red, but it disappeared within hours and I was fine. It was wonderful to know that I could add facials back into my life. The more normal things I can do, the more like myself I feel."

If you go in for a facial, you may have to take charge, even if the person claims to know how to treat rosacea skin. If you sense that what is on your face is going to irritate it, then ask to have it removed. If the cloth on your face is too hot, ask that it be cooled down. And don't buy any products. If the person is truly knowl-edgeable about rosacea, they won't try to sell you anything, knowing there is a good chance you could react adversely to it. Instead, you should be offered a sample of a product to try at home. If it's not offered, ask for it. And if the first aesthetician doesn't meet your needs, then try another one. If the next facial still aggravates your skin, it may mean you need to wait until your rosacea is under better control.

Products to Improve the Texture of Your Skin

Facial rejuvenation seems to be the new buzzword these days— everybody wants their skin to look younger. Even without rosacea, years of sun exposure will damage anyone's skin. While some products used to diminish the appearance of wrinkles, such as Retin-A, are far too irritating for people with rosacea, new products are coming to the market that may be possible for you to use. An example of this is a treatment called Kinerase. Available over the counter, it comes in lotion and cream forms, depending on your skin type (oily or dry). Kinerase doesn't cause burning or tingling, so it's not likely to bother your skin (although with rosacea, there are no 100 percent guarantees). Kinerase does not thin the skin, which is a definite plus with rosacea, and it is both hypoallergenic and noncomedogenic. The manufacturers claim it reduces fine wrinkles, improves skin texture, and fades hyper-pigmentation (brown spots).

Topical vitamin C is said to also improve the appearance of sun damaged skin. The claim is that it will increase collagen pro-duction, improve elasticity and firmness, and reduce fine lines and wrinkles. Since vitamin C has strong antioxidant properties, it will also protect the skin from environmental stresses. The problem is that many people with rosacea have found vitamin C products to be irritating to their skin. It may be the form of the vitamin C itself or the base that it's formulated in. There may be a way around this, however: Mary The, an aesthetician in San Francisco, uses a product that has vitamin C in the non-acidic form of magnesium ascorbyl phosphate. She has found it to be healing and soothing to the skin of those with rosacea.

These types of products allow those with rosacea to also have access to the current rage of anti-aging products, and provide one more tool for improving the appearance of your face.

Microdermabrasion

If you want to take your facial rejuvenation even further, microdermabrasion may be a possibility for you. Some with rosacea may have problems with this procedure, but others tolerate it well. The procedure involves a fine stream of crystal particles, which are sprayed on the face to gently remove superficial skin, layer by layer, until new skin cells appear. The claim is that this gentle exfoliation restores healthy skin texture, reducing fine lines and wrinkles, cleaning away blackheads, removing age spots, reducing minor scars, and decreasing pore size.

Alan is a fifty-two-year-old man who has had microdermabrasion about four times. "I was hesitant at first, but I really like it. There is no discomfort and I like the way it makes my skin look. At first, I was a little red, but I experimented and took an aspirin about an hour before, which seems to have prevented any inflammation. Also, the woman that does my treatments rolls these balls that have been dipped in cold water over my face when we're done, and it's incredibly soothing. I'm sure it helps minimize the flushing. I also bring my own moisturizer to apply after the treatment, because I know it works well for me. I really think the appearance of my face is improving. My skin is usually so dry, but the microdermabrasion, since it exfoliates, makes it look much better. What I especially like is that I see a decrease in pore size, which really makes me happy. I just hate that orange peel appearance that sometimes occurs with enlarged pores."

Treating Telangiectasias

The goal in your everyday approach to controlling rosacea is generally to prevent flaring—to keep the redness down and to prevent the breakouts. Through appropriate dietary control, nutritional supplements, and various topical treatments, you will eventually gain the upper hand. But what about those red lines that traverse your face? Maybe the appearance of new vessels has slowed dramatically, but they occasionally still occur. You may also have prominent capillaries that dilated unbecomingly before you even knew you had rosacea.

Pulsed Dye Lasers

There are many different types of lasers being used today for various medical conditions. The application for a particular laser is determined by its specific wavelength and power output. The pulsed dye laser has been used for many years to treat the telangiectasias of rosacea. Here's how it works: When the laser is directed at the skin, the light energy is absorbed by various pigments, the important pigment in the case of rosacea being hemoglobin. As the light is absorbed by the damaged blood vessels, they are heated, sealed, and eventually reabsorbed into the body.

The pulsed dye laser produces yellow light, which is better absorbed by hemoglobin than any other color. The pulsed dye laser produces good results, but you'll end up looking like you went a few rounds with Muhammad Ali. For at least a week, your face will be covered with large purple bruises. This will often not be just a one-time treatment, because until you get control of your rosacea, you may produce more dilated, damaged, and leaky capillaries. So you have to decide how many times you are willing to go through this. It takes a brave soul to venture out in public with this appearance, but for some it's worth it.

Modern treatments do bring their own coping challenges. Arlene, fifty, a lifelong Connecticut resident, began receiving laser treatments on her cheeks in her mid-forties. She had suffered from rosacea outbreaks since passing through a rather early menopause. "I call it my Pippie Longstocking look," she laughs, referring to the wine-colored spots on her cheeks, resembling huge freckles, that appeared after treatment. "For a week or more I would hide in a dark bedroom. If I absolutely had to venture out, I would wear a balaclava, which hid the spots but made me look like an international terrorist." The difficulty of dealing with the aftermath of treatment was a factor in convincing her to try the gentler intense pulsed light (IPL) approach to ameliorating her rosacea symptoms.

Intense Pulsed Light

So what exactly is IPL? More commonly called PhotoDerm, after the device that is used for the procedure, it is the newest machinery in the fight against the dilated capillaries and flushing of rosacea. It is a laserlike device that puts out intense light and allows the operator of the machine to set the device precisely for each individual's skin, allowing exact treatment of the dilated vessels and redness. The beauty of this is that even the tiniest and deepest vessels can be treated, yet the surrounding skin is not harmed. The difference between laser treatment and this intense light treatment is that the laser, since it only produces a single wavelength of light, is limited to how deeply it penetrates and what it can treat. The PhotoDerm machine emits light that produces many wavelengths, thus allowing penetration to all levels of skin where abnormal vessels can be found.

Besides decreasing facial flushing and eliminating the appearance of dilated capillaries, treatment with the PhotoDerm also has the pleasant side effect of generally improving appearance of your skin. People have noticed a decrease in pore size, a lessening of fine wrinkles, and an increase in skin smoothness. This is due to the fact that the intense light generates new collagen formation, which gives the skin a more youthful appearance.

Each treatment takes between twenty minutes and an hour, depending on the practitioner and the needs of the patient. To make the procedure bearable, insist that a topical anesthetic be applied about a half hour before treatment. It will still be uncomfortable, but with the topical treatment, it's tolerable.

What's especially nice is that you leave the office with only a red face, which seems to respond well and quickly to an ice pack. By the evening, or certainly the next day, many people are no longer flushed from the treatment. It is possible to bruise or blister, but such a reaction is rare.

The recommended protocol is a series of five treatments at intervals of three to four weeks. At this time, it is anticipated that people will need a touch-up treatment every one to two years, depending on the individual. But keep in mind that this is a new therapy, so it is hard to know exactly how often touch-ups will be required. Jerry, thirty-six, is thrilled with his response to the PhotoDerm treatment. "My overall flushing has been reduced by 80 to 90 percent. And without the flushing I no longer suffer from a severely burning face. As a result, I can use sunblocks and other topical products for the first time in years."

When a new technique comes along, lots of practitioners will jump on the bandwagon without being properly trained. So, as with any type of procedure, it's important to thoroughly investigate who will be treating you. Ask where they learned the treatment and how many people they have treated. If you're at all uneasy, ask if they would be willing to give you the names of people they have treated so that you can talk to them personally. You might also want to get on a rosacea board on the Internet and ask if anyone has had experience with the office you're considering. This is true not just for the PhotoDerm procedure but for any type of laser treatment.

Debby, age thirty-eight, learned a lesson firsthand about the minefield of treatments and practitioners out there. About eight years ago she decided that she wanted to do something about the telangiectasias on her cheeks and nose, because she had become very self-conscious about them. She was about to see a dermatologist, but a close friend, a physician, suggested that she instead see a plastic surgeon, because after all, it was her face she was talking about. She saw the surgeon, and he set her up with his nurse, who gave her two laser treatments. After the second treatment Debby noticed pitting on her cheeks. In panic, she went back to the office, and the nurse told her the pitting was due to her skin type and she could no longer have any treatment for her dilated capillaries. She would just have to live with them for the rest of her life. Debby was not told that there were any other types of laser treatments available.

She was depressed for months, until one day she read about the pulsed dye laser. She went to talk to a dermatologist, and although he was careful in what he said, she was smart enough to figure it out for herself. "What I realized is that the plastic surgeon's office had an old-type laser that they owned and were determined to keep using. What is unconscionable is that once it had adverse affects on me, they blamed me for it, and let me think that there were no other options out there." She adds, "What I liked about the dermatologist is that he didn't own the pulsed dye laser machine—he only rented it. To me, that meant if he found something better, his medical judgment wouldn't be based on the economics of keeping a machine just because he'd paid for it already."

Investigate New Lasers

As technology continues to advance, you'll hear about new devices and treatments. Already, for example, two new lasers, Versapulse and V-beam, are being used to treat those tiny visible blood vessels. They are less painful than the older pulsed dye laser, and they cause no bruising, which means no downtime. You can get back to your normal life immediately after the treatment. The important thing is to be cautious and do your own research on the procedures and the people performing them. It can be confusing when each doctor you see explains why his or her particular treatment is the state of the art. It's unfortunate, but many doctors have a financial reason for touting their particular machine. You need to always keep this fact in mind, and you also have to keep in mind that your particular symptomatology (maybe you flush all over, or maybe you just have visible superficial vessels) may benefit most from a particular type of treatment

Although the best course of treatment may be difficult to determine, we are enormously lucky to be living in a time where the worst side effects of rosacea can be treated. You don't need to panic over permanently dilated capillaries, because they can be treated effectively. And rhinophyma (the red and bumpy nose of rosacea) can be treated. One type of laser can remove the visible blood vessels, and another type of laser can be used to remove the excess tissue and reshape the nose. All this is wonderful news that should provide relief for people with rosacea.

The not-so-good news is that the different laser and light treatments are rarely covered by insurance (see appendix). In their arbitrary way, insurance companies see this as an unnecessary cosmetic procedure. They don't understand that these therapies are vital for the emotional and subsequent physical health of someone with rosacea. And, unfortunately, there's nobody out there fighting this battle for us. Hopefully, as time goes on, the procedures will become less expensive as there is more utilization of this new technology and more competition between providers.

7

Nutrition for Your Skin

Your skin is in constant contact with the environment around you, and no doubt you, are already well aware of how various substances, ranging from fabrics and household products, to cosmetics, soaps, lotions, affect your skin. In fact, it's hard to imagine any organ of your body (your skin *is* an organ, after all) having more contact with your environment than your skin. There is, however, another critically important organ system that is in very intimate contact with a huge part of your environment. We're talking about your intestinal tract, and the part of your environment we're referring to is what you eat and drink every day. On average, you swallow up to a ton of food and drink each year, and all of it is in direct contact with you for many hours, even days, while it is being filtered, processed, and absorbed. Wonderful nutrients or harmful substances—whichever you take in—then get delivered to all parts of your body, including your skin.

Although this chapter is about nutrition for your skin, it's important to remember that your body is a whole, integrated system in which all of the parts and functions are interconnected. Whatever provides benefit or harm to your skin therefore affects the rest of your body. In fact, the overall health of your body may well be reflected in the health of your skin.

There are many foods, herbs, and supplemental nutrients that are beneficial for your skin, as well as foods and substances that can be harmful. This is true even for those who don't have rosacea. In order to keep yourself and your skin healthy and vibrant, it is most important to take in nourishing, wholesome food each day. Nature has provided a cornucopia of treasures for you to use to keep yourself looking wonderful and feeling good.

So Many Kinds of Dietary Theories

In the last several years, all kinds of recommendations for the perfect diet have been put forth. You may well have heard of a number of them. There is the Ornish Diet, the Pritikin Diet, the McDougall Plan, the Atkins Diet, the Zone Diet, the Metabolic Typing Diet, the Blood Type Diet, the Carbohydrate Addict's Diet ... and that's just to name a few. While each of these dietary approaches has been reported to benefit a number of people, there are deeper, more fundamental truths about the kinds of foods that have nourished extraordinarily healthy and long-lived cultures of people for millennia. It is from this perspective that we offer our recommendations for healthy nutrition to benefit your skin.

Foods, Herbs, and Nutrients Your Skin Will Like

The foods, herbs, and nutrients listed below are those that we feel promote the health of your entire body, including your skin. This list is meant to give you an overview of the kinds of foods we believe are most nourishing. However, even among the foods that are normally considered wholesome and healthy, there may be those that your body doesn't like. You may have found that you are allergic or sensitive to certain of these foods, or that one or more of them trigger your rosacea. If that's the case, you would of course want to avoid them. You may want to keep a journal or use the Rosacea Diary Checklist in chapter 4 to see if you can trace which foods may be causing you to experience a flare-up. There are enough varieties of wonderful foods available that you will still have plenty of options in each of the categories represented here.

As a general guideline for daily amounts, having 20 to 30 percent of your calories as protein foods, 25 to 30 percent as fats and oils, and 45 to 55 percent as carbohydrate foods, primarily in the form of vegetables and some fruits, is a good place to start. You may want to adjust these amounts to accommodate your particular needs. Try to get fresh, organically grown foods and herbs (or at least try to get them free from herbicides, pesticides, fungicides, antibiotics, and hormones if at all possible). If organic or unsprayed foods are not available to you, just get the freshest ones you can. If you can't get fresh, then buy them frozen. Frozen foods still retain a lot more of their nutrients than canned, but if all else fails, better canned than none.

Foods

* Lots of vegetables—30 to 35 percent of caloric intake would look like about 60 to 65 percent of your food, if you were to lay it all out on a tabletop.

* Include liberal use of garlic and onions (also listed as herbs, below).

* Small amounts of organic or contaminant-free seaweeds (if available).

* Moderate amounts of fresh fruits (equivalent to one to two servings per day), preferably in season.

* Animal protein—including fish, poultry, moderate amounts of meat, and eggs; also (if tolerated) cultured dairy products, such as certified organic, raw milk cheeses, yogurt, and kefir from goat, sheep, or cow sources.

* Whole grains, prepared so that their inherent digestion-inhibiting properties (Reinhold 1972) are reduced or eliminated. (See chapter 9 to learn this technique.) You might want to try either low-gluten grains, such as amaranth and quinoa, or grains that contain a slightly different form of gluten (gliadin-free), such as brown/red/black rices, millet, or corn. Wheat, rye, oats, and barley are the highest in the kind of gluten that contains gliadin, which is the particular protein found in gluten that has been found to create both clinical gluten

intolerance (celiac disease) and sub-clinical gluten intolerance, which can manifest as a variety of systemic inflammatory conditions.

✳ Beans, also ideally prepared to reduce their phytates and enzyme-inhibiting properties. (See chapter 9.)

✳ Nuts, such as almonds, walnuts, hazelnuts; seeds such as sunflower seeds and sesame seeds. Flax seeds may have particular benefits (see chapter 8).

✳ Stone-crushed, cold pressed, extra virgin olive oil.

✳ Avocados—a natural source of monounsaturated fat.

✳ Small amounts of organic, untoasted sesame oil.

✳ Moderate amounts of cultured organic butter.

✳ Ghee (clarified butter) and/or organic coconut butter for sautéing.

✳ Celtic sea salt, or other natural, unprocessed sea salt.

Beverages

We have one word for you here: water. Drinking plenty of fresh water is so often overlooked and so important. You've heard for years that you should drink at least six to eight glasses of water each day. This is a good guideline, but remember that when you include lots of fresh vegetables and a reasonable amount of fresh fruits, you don't need as much water, because these foods contain a significant amount of natural water.

Nutrients in Supplement Form

One important point to make here before listing any supplements is that it is essential that you get as much nutrient value from your food as you possibly can. Many sources agree that nutritional supplements can be very helpful and supportive for overall health and the health of your skin, but there are hundreds of thousands of nutrients in food that cannot be duplicated in any supplement. So, it is important to keep in mind that your supplements are there to do just that—*supplement* the nutrients in your food, not replace them. We also believe it is important for you to get top quality supplements, so don't be afraid to ask questions and get as much information as you can as you make your selections.

According to one source, the Recommended Daily Allowance (RDA) for vitamins and minerals was devised to prevent deficiency diseases resulting from malnutrition, rather than support total wellness by meeting optimal nutritional needs (Murray 1996). This is why many nutritionally oriented professionals recommend amounts that are often significantly greater than the RDA. Since fresh whole foods do contain most of these nutrients, the amounts of any additional nutrients that you might take in supplement form would ideally be adjusted to complement and augment what you take in through your food. This can be rather tricky to determine. As you may have already noticed, if you've examined the labels of multivitamin/multimineral formulas, the amounts usually given are frequently offered as though you wouldn't be getting any of these nutrients from your food. In light of all this, although we recommend higher amounts of nutrients than the RDA, the amounts we are suggesting are somewhat conservative. Be sure you see your health care practitioner if you have particular health issues or are taking medications, and you are planning to take supplements. With this in mind, here are some general suggestions.

Vitamins & Minerals	Suggested Daily Amounts
❋ Natural vitamin A—in cod liver oil	5000–7000 IU (see note below with cautions for pregnant women)
❋ Vitamin C—nonacidic ascorbate form	500–1500 mg
❋ Vitamin E—in base of mixed beta gamma, and delta tocopherols	400 IU d-alpha tocopherol
❋ Natural vitamin D—in cod liver oil	400—800 IU
❋ B-complex vitamins—well balanced, carefully manufactured, and hypo-allergenic if possible), including:	
Thiamine (B_1)	25–100 mg
Riboflavin (B_2)	20–50 mg

Niacinamide(B$_3$) or	10–20 mg/
Inositol hexaniacinate	30–50mg
(nonflushing form of niacin)	
Pantothenic acid (B$_5$)	25–100 mg
Pyridoxine HCL (B$_6$)	25–100 mg
Biotin	300 mcg
B$_{12}$	400–800 mcg
Folic acid	400–800 mcg

❋ Multimineral formula, well balanced and properly chelated, using, for example, the Albion Laboratories chelation process; chelates like citrate, malate, ascorbate, glycinate, lysinate, and taurinate have a reputation for better absorbability than the carbonate or oxide forms:

Calcium	500–1000 mg
Magnesium—approx.	500–1000 mg
1:1 ratio to calcium	
Manganese	10–20 mg
Boron	1–5 mg
Zinc	10–20 mg
Copper—about 1:10 ratio to zinc	1–2 mg
Selenium	100–200 mcg
Chromium	100–300 mcg
Molybdenum	50–100 mcg
Vanadium	50–100 mcg

A note on vitamin A and pregnancy: According to Zand and Spreen (1999), pregnant women should not ingest more than 25,000 IU per week from all sources. Balch and Balch (1997) recommend that pregnant women not exceed 10,000 IU per day.

You'll notice that iron in supplement form isn't listed here, as it can build up in your system and contribute to your body's free radical load, and even suppress your immune system. (Free radicals are molecules that can cause DNA damage and are potentially carcinogenic). Iron is an essential nutrient, however, and is readily available from whole foods. Your body's ability to make good use of it depends upon an adequate supply of other nutrients such as the minerals listed above and vitamin C. If you are truly low in iron, you should see your health care provider.

Also, iodine isn't listed since it may, according to some reports, exacerbate skin eruptions (Hitch 1967). However it is essential for proper thyroid function, and you can obtain all you need from natural sources, such as fish and seaweed. Iodized salt contains iodine as well, but this iodine is not in a natural form. You may want to switch to a natural, unprocessed sea salt or Celtic sea salt, both of which contain traces of not only natural iodine but dozens of other beneficial, although less well known, trace minerals.

Additional Supplements and Antioxidants	Suggested Daily Amounts
❈ Cod liver oil—extracted from healthy fish, and carefully produced to avoid oxidation and heavy metal contamination; not to exceed upper limits for vitamins A & D.	½–1 tsp liquid or 1–3 softgels
❈ EPA and DHA omega–3 fatty acids.	EPA: 360–1080 mg DHA: 240–720 mg
❈ Flax seed oil—source of plant-based omega-3 acid	½–1 tsp
❈ GLA derivative of omega–6 fatty acid—borage oil is the richest source.	240–720 mg
❈ MSM (methylsulfonyl-methane) has shown anti-inflammatory effects (Mindell 1997).	500–1000 mg
❈ Probiotics such as acidophilus and bifido bacteria—for intestinal health, essential to restore beneficial intestinal bacteria, especially necessary after antibiotic treatment (Mercola 1999).	Take as directed on bottle.
❈ Plant-based digestive enzymes.	Take as directed on bottle.
❈ Betaine hydrochloride supplements.	Take as directed with protein.
❈ Mixed carotenoids—includes alpha and beta carotenes, lutein, zeaxanthin,	10,000–15,000 IU

cryptoxanthin, rather than only beta
carotene isolated from the rest.

✳ Bioflavonoids—thousands occur   50–500 mg each
naturally in vegetables and fruits;
a few have been isolated for
supplementation, such as PCO
(proanthocyanidin, also known as
pycnogenol, also known as GSE
[grapeseed extract, *not to be confused
with grapefruit seed extract, which is also
called GSE*]), anthocyanidins, catechins,
ellagic acid, hesperidin, rutin, etc.;
PCO (GSE) and rutin have capillary-
strengthening and anti-inflammatory
effects (Keville 1995 and Murray 1996).

✳ Quercetin—anti-inflammatory,   250–500 mg
occurs naturally in onion and garlic.

✳ Bromelain—pineapple enzyme   500–2000 mg
concentrate, a potent anti-inflammatory.

Culinary Herbs

Culinary herbs are the ones that are commonly used in cooking to flavor our foods. These wonderful culinary herbs are not
only delicious, but they offer other properties including natural
antioxidant activity (ao), anti-microbial activity for a healthy
intestinal tract (am), a calming effect (cm), and even skin healing
(sk) (Holmes 1994). They can be found either fresh or recently
dried and packaged. The primary way you can tell if herbs have
been "sitting around forever" is by smell. The smell will either be
very weak, or have a "stale" quality, or may even smell a bit like
urine. The secondary way is that the color of the herb will appear
muted, perhaps brownish or grayish in color, rather than a fresh
green (or whatever color is natural to the part of the herb being
used, such as the berry, root, or stem).

Try to find unsprayed herbs if you can. You may even enjoy
growing your own herbs in containers, and either using them
fresh, or drying them by cutting and bunching them (separately)
and hanging them upside down in a dark, dry place until they've
dried. Then you can crumble them into little glass jars and—

voila!—you've got your own homemade dried herbs to flavor your foods and add wonderful healing nutrients to your daily diet.

❈ Basil (am, cm)   ❈ Marjoram (cm)   ❈ Oregano (am, cm)

❈ Rosemary (ao, am)   ❈ Sage (am, sk)   ❈ Tarragon (ao, am)

❈ Thyme (ao, am)

Anti-inflammatory Herbs

Certain herbs have a history of being used as extracts, dried powders, or teas to support healthy skin because of their anti-inflammatory properties (i.e., calming down systemic inflammation and, in some cases, even preventing it altogether). All have been used to help reduce inflammation of the skin as well (Lininger et al. 1998).

Medicinal Herbs

❈ Aloe vera   ❈ Boswellia   ❈ Burdock root

❈ Chickweed   ❈ Coleus forskohlii   ❈ Dandelion leaf/root

❈ Nettle leaf   ❈ Red clover flower   ❈ Red beet root

❈ Stillengia herb   ❈ Turmeric (curcumin)   ❈ Yarrow

❈ Yellow dock   ❈ Yucca

Herbs for Reducing Capillary Fragility
(Pederson 1994; Lininger et al. 1998; Holmes 1994)

❈ Bilberry   ❈ Butcher's broom   ❈ Gotu kola

❈ Rose hips fruit   ❈ Horse chestnut extract

❈ Grape seed extract (Murray 1996)

Herbs for Liver Support and Intestinal Health

In addition, there are some wonderful herbs that offer particular support for your liver in its constant job of detoxifying the daily barrage of substances that come to it (Galland 1997). Supporting your liver helps to keep internal toxins from circulating throughout your body, where they can build up in various tissues, including your skin (Cabot 1999). A toxin is defined as any compound that has a detrimental effect on cell function or structure. Toxins can include toxic chemicals (such as solvents, drugs, alcohol, pesticides, herbicides, food additives), heavy metals (such as lead, mercury, cadmium, arsenic, nickel, and aluminum), microbial compounds (waste products and cellular debris from bacteria and yeast in the intestines, known as endotoxins), and breakdown products of protein metabolism (such as ammonia, urea, etc.). Many of these come through, or are created within, your own intestinal tract (Galland 1997 and Nolan 1989). They are passed on to your liver, and can overload your liver and circulate systemically, becoming irritants to your skin. We'll cover this more thoroughly in chapter 9. Many of the herbs that support your liver also directly benefit the health of your intestinal tract.

✳ Aloe vera   ✳ Artichoke leaf   ✳ Burdock root

✳ Dandelion   ✳ Fennel   ✳ Garlic

✳ Green tea (unless you're avoiding caffeine completely)

✳ Marshmallow root   ✳ Milk thistle   ✳ Onion

✳ Pau d'arco bark   ✳ Picrorhiza root   ✳ Red clover

✳ Slippery elm bark   ✳ Turmeric (curcumin)

Relaxing and Calming Herbs

Some herbs are relaxing and calming in general—not specifically as anti-inflammatories or as sedatives, but as overall soothers of your nervous system, endocrine system, and perhaps even your psyche, all of which helps your skin (Holmes 1994).

These herbs can frequently be found as teas, either individually or in combination with other herbs. Many companies are now offering certified organically grown teas. In one study, chamomile was reported to have anti-inflammatory activity when applied topically (Tubaro 1984).

✳ Chamomile   ✳ Lemon balm (melissa)   ✳ Spearmint

✳ Valerian root

Tips for Herb Use

Many of the herbs we've listed, both culinary and medicinal, are now available as organic, or unsprayed and nonirradiated. If possible, try to find herbs that are prepared as "whole" herbs, rather than extractions of only the acknowledged "potent" factor(s). Herbal preparations have been prepared for millennia from whole herbs. Only in more recent decades have the herbs been dissected, so to speak, in order to isolate and concentrate the particular components that science has decided are the important ones.

While there are certain factors in all herbs that seem to provide the benefits we're looking for, these "desirable" factors work synergistically with the other components of the whole herb, components that may not be known or understood yet. Using whole herb products assures that all the synergistic factors are present.

If you find that any amount of alcohol can trigger a rosacea flare-up, you will not want to use alcohol-based herbal extracts. The best process for preparing herbs is probably the one perfected by Eclectic Institute of Sandy, Oregon. They prepare most of their herbs by freeze-drying the whole herb, crumbling it to a powder, and presenting it in capsule form. This preserves all the natural factors in the herbs, including all those that would be destroyed by heat or alcohol. Second best is the process of extracting the whole herb and presenting it in a non-alcohol glycerol base. This doesn't preserve the natural factors nearly to the degree that freeze-drying does, but does offer an alternative to the freeze-dried type. Eclectic Institute, Herb Pharm, Rainbow Light, and Gaia offer various herbal extracts in this form.

If you have difficulty finding products by these companies in your area, then just do the best you can. If you are hooked up to the Internet, you may be able to access many products that way. You may also be able to find many of these herbs as teas. In this case, you can brew them just as you would any tea, unless there are special instructions on the package. Herbs sold in capsules or liquid extracts (i.e., in bottles or packages) are best taken in the dosages that are recommended on the label unless you are under the care of a health care practitioner who may have specific recommendations for you.

Foods and Drinks Your Skin Doesn't Like

Now we come to the information about foods and drinks that either *don't* nourish your skin or can actually be stressful to it. As a point of clarity, what will be listed here are the actual foods themselves, as distinguished from the hundreds of chemicals, including pesticides, herbicides, fungicides, preservatives, flavor enhancers, artificial colorings, etc., which end up in our food supply, but are not actually part of the food itself. Of course it's important to avoid as much of this chemical onslaught as possible, because it is becoming widely recognized that these chemicals are contributing to increasing stress on our immune systems, and can, in and of themselves, trigger inflammation of the skin or any other tissue of the body. (More about this in chapter 8.) For now, though, it's the actual foods themselves to which we are referring.

Skin Stressors

The first group lists foods and drinks that are on many different "avoid" lists because of their reputation for stressing and even weakening all systems of the body. Since the skin is an excretory organ, it can become irritated as it tries to eliminate certain components of these foods and drinks that your body sees as undesirable.

Unfortunately, some of the items in this first group are things that many of us tend to love. Here's a comforting thought, though: Once you get used to not having these things, and you shift over more and more to healing, nourishing, and regenerative foods and drinks, believe it or not, your craving for the "forbidden" stressful ones will begin to weaken. These are foods that can stress or weaken your skin and your entire system:

❋ Alcohol   ❋ Coffee

❋ Sugar   ❋ Refined carbohydrates (sugar in disguise)

❋ Overheated/rancid/hydrogenated/partially hydrogenated fats and oils

❋ Chlorinated water

Allergic Reactions

As you read in chapter 4, there are a number of foods that have been reported to cause a histamine response, which can exacerbate your rosacea. This production of histamine is created by your immune system's production of IgE immunoglobulin.

And when it happens in response to eating certain foods, it is defined by allergists as a true food allergy, as differentiated from a food sensitivity or intolerance (Marinkovich 1999).

Janine a veterinarian from Colorado, was affected by histamine reactions. She had been raised in a health conscious household, and always ate fresh fruits in the summertime. "I always looked forward to summer. Even though I have to be careful of the heat, so my rosacea doesn't act up, I've always felt good in the summer. We always had fresh fruits, especially strawberries, my favorite. A couple of summers ago I started having more problems with my face breaking out. I thought maybe it was the sunscreen I was using, so I stopped using it. It didn't get better; it got worse. I finally realized that the breakouts were happening within an hour or two after I would indulge in my favorite fruit. No way, I thought—they weren't on my 'avoid' list! Was I imagining this? I had to see if it was true. I stopped eating the strawberries and the next day my face started calming right down. I was devastated at first. But, through necessity, I started trying some of the new exotic fruits in the market. I now have three favorites instead of just one. And none of them affect my face."

The following foods have been reported to cause histamine response—the formation of IgE antibodies, called true food allergy (Murray and Pizzorno 1998):

- avocado
- bananas
- cheese
- citrus
- chocolate
- chicken eggs
- nuts, especially peanuts
- shellfish
- tomatoes
- tuna (canned)
- vinegar
- yogurt

Food Sensitivities and Intolerances

Dr. Leo Galland, M.D., a clinician and author in New York City who specializes in diseases that are hard to diagnose or treat, includes rosacea in his list of disorders in which specific food allergies or food intolerances are frequently encountered (and have often gone unsuspected) (1997).

Some foods may create problems not because you are allergic to them, but because they may irritate your intestinal lining and not digest thoroughly. This can lead to the formation of immune complexes, which primarily involves IgG immunoglobulins.

These complexes can circulate to your skin, where they cause inflammation and put you at risk for a flare-up.

According to Dr. Vincent Marinkovich, M.D., specialist in allergy/immunology at Stanford Medical School, when you eat a food to which you develop significant antibody levels, molecules of these foods can pass through the intestinal wall without being completely digested, and combine with your immune system's antibodies, usually IgG antibodies, to form immune complexes that circulate around in the body. If too many of these immune complexes are formed, your body cannot remove them all from circulation, and they tend to deposit in various tissues. Wherever they end up, they create inflammatory conditions that lead to illness focused upon that particular organ. "We tend to make antibodies in a pattern, ourselves, depending upon our inherited ability to do that. Therefore, we differ from one another in how we respond to a single food. So, there are various consequences of immune complex deposition in tissues where they can cause illness that depends upon the kind of overwhelm or breakdown of the body's normal system for removing these complexes successfully and peacefully from the circulation" (1999).

In terms of people suffering from rosacea, Dr. Marinkovich thinks that these patients all have an overload of immune complexes, probably from foods, but possibly from chronic infection. Once you reach an overload, you can't clear these complexes quickly from your circulation, so they tend to float around. When they reach the skin, it's cooler than the internal body temperature, especially the face, since it's exposed rather than covered by clothing. However, he says, "remember that we haven't done any studies with rosacea, so what I'm saying about rosacea is largely just speculative, but it is within the context of sound immunological science" (Marinkovich 2000).

Most of what is on the following food sensitivity list will not surprise you, since many of these items are also included in published rosacea "trigger" lists. Interestingly, you may have already noticed that certain foods that either cause or intensify your flare-ups don't appear on any of the published trigger lists. This doesn't mean that you've been imagining your reactions, or that your system is somehow abnormal. The fact is that although we are all physiologically and biochemically similar, our genes make us unique, so that each of us is to a certain degree an exception to the "rule." In other words, no one is genetically exactly the same as you (unless you have an identical twin!). When you consider the countless combinations of factors that constitute *you*, and consider that no one else has your exact combination of factors, you can understand that you truly are unique. So, don't be surprised if the particular foods and drinks that trigger a flare-up for you aren't on the standard trigger lists. The following foods have been reported to cause delayed food intolerance or sensitivity reactions (formation of IgG antibodies):

* wheat products

* gluten grains other than wheat: rye, oats, barley, spelt, kamut, amaranth

* conventional cow dairy products

* soy products: soy milk, tofu, soy protein isolate (read labels)

* pork

* beef

Testing for Food Allergies or Sensitivities

There are self-tests that you can use to help you learn which foods your system reacts to unfavorably. We'll briefly describe just a couple of them here. One is called the pulse test. The evidence to support this test is purely anecdotal, but you may want to give it a try. In a resting state, you take your pulse and record it. Then by itself, you eat the food you are testing. Record your pulse again, at several intervals—ten minutes, twenty minutes, one hour, one and a half hours, two hours, and even three hours. If your pulse has increased by ten or more beats per minute, *assuming that nothing else has changed significantly that would affect your pulse,* you can assume that you are having a negative response to that food.

The best method of self-testing is the elimination/challenge diet. There are a number of different suggestions for doing this. One recommendation is to make a list of foods that you eat daily, or that you crave, and that you suspect make you feel bad. According to some authorities, foods with a very high allergy or sensitivity potential are bread and other wheat products, milk and other dairy products, eggs, citrus fruits, and their juices, chocolate, corn, soy products, peanut products, tomatoes, and yeast.

Eliminate the foods on your list for seven to fourteen days, recording any changes you may experience. You can then bring back, one at a time, each food you omitted. Every four or five days, bring back another food from your list, and record any reactions. This takes a number of weeks or even months to do, but often can reveal the very foods that may be stimulating your immune system into action and even triggering a direct or delayed rosacea outbreak.

Something you might want to consider is rotating your foods so that you aren't eating the same foods day after day (Lipski 2000). One suggestion is to rotate your foods every four days. This will encourage you to bring more variety into your diet, which, according to some authorities, may lessen the possibility that your immune system will build up an unfavorable reaction to the foods you eat. Diversifying can become an adventure: The world has gotten smaller, and we now have access to a whole array of enticing, tasty choices that can bring both pleasure and good health.

If you are interested in other available testing modalities, see our Web site (www.rosaceaworld.com) for additional resources.

8

What You Eat

What Do We Mean by "Good Nutrition"?

The concept of good nutrition has been around for a long time, and what it actually means can be described in a number of ways, depending on your philosophy of health care. Suffice it to say that we do not subscribe to the prevailing medical view of nutrition. We believe that optimum health requires much more care and discrimination in selecting the foods and nutrients we put into our bodies. Good nutrition simply means choosing foods that truly serve you, foods that are naturally rich in valuable nutrients and are free from harmful chemicals, foods that best support vibrant health. It also means eating and drinking these foods in such a way that all the tissues of your body (and in your case, especially your skin) actually receive the valuable nutrients instead of receiving harmful toxins from inadequately digested foods and an unhealthy balance of intestinal flora (Bland 1999). (We'll go into this more thoroughly in chapter 9.)

How Important Is Organic Food?

We feel compelled to emphasize the importance of organically raised foods for two reasons. First, certified organic foods are free from pesticide residues. There is increasing evidence that conventionally raised foods, which may contain residues of herbicides, pesticides, fungicides, and hormone substances, and are processed with additives and preservatives, contribute to the increasing array of degenerative diseases many of us suffer today. Some researchers are finding that the chemicals that continue to make their way into our foodstuffs are overloading and even disabling our immune systems (Percival 1999). Secondly, the soils used in organic farming are free of damaging chemicals and are richer in organic matter and soil microorganisms, which process soil minerals into forms that the plants can readily uptake, resulting in foods that contain higher levels of nutrients. This has been shown in various studies (Rateaver and Rateaver 1973; Rodale Institute 1997). Organically raised foods have been shown to be richer in natural minerals, vitamins, antioxidants, and other valuable nutrients than conventionally grown foods (Pizzorno 1996).

Organic food is the ideal, but unfortunately it is generally more expensive than conventional supermarket food, unless you can find a good farmers' market. Also, even if you may prefer to buy organic food, it may not be easy or even possible to get it, depending on where you live. If organic is not an option for you, don't despair—all is not lost. We believe organic foods are optimal, but the choice is ultimately yours.

What are your options? Just keep the phrase "clean and simple" in mind. This means that even if you can't buy organic, you should buy foods that are fresh and unprocessed, as close to their "natural" state as possible. If you are in an area where you have seasonal access to locally grown foods, by all means take advantage of these foods. They will be fresher and more nutritious than anything you can buy in a supermarket.

It's important to wash all produce, but if your produce is conventional, it is particularly important to wash it carefully to remove as much chemical residue as you can. There are a number of recommendations for doing this. One is to use a mixture of a quarter-cup vinegar in one gallon of warm water, which may accelerate the breakdown of some pesticides (Gittleman 1999). Another is to use a solution of one teaspoon of bleach to one gallon of water; soak leafy vegetables and thin-skinned fruits for fifteen minutes and root-type, fibrous, or thick-skinned vegetables and fruits for thirty minutes. There are also produce cleansing products that are primarily derived from coconut, such as VegiWash or EarthSafe. For organic produce, where you are removing only some soil and soil bacteria, you can use the same solutions for shorter periods of time.

Again, the emphasis is on: 1) *what* you choose to eat and drink and 2) *how* you eat and drink these things.

Our Basic Guidelines for Good Nutrition

❋ Eat simply. The less "processed" your food is, the better for you.

❋ Whenever possible, eat certified organically grown foods. If you can't get organically grown foods, try to find foods free from pesticides, herbicides, fungicides, antibiotics, hormones, etc. Thousands of potentially harmful chemicals can be avoided just by doing this alone. If you can't obtain either, buy foods that are as fresh and natural as possible.

❋ Eat a healthy balance of foods (more on this below).

❋ Eat the RIGHT fats and oils (see below).

❋ Make sure the foods you eat are thoroughly and completely digested (see chapter 9).

Saving Your Face: WHAT You Eat and Drink

There are certain nutritional requirements that all of us have in common. There are also certain foods and substances that many have experienced as being difficult to digest, or harmful, or both.

While it's important to know what we all have in common, and it is just as important to know how we differ. You are unique. What may be beneficial and healing to someone else may be seen as harmful by your own individual immune system, and vice versa. Finding out what foods serve you best, and what foods provide the most nutrients with the least amount of stress on your immune system is key to maximizing your body's potential to heal and stay well. This is crucial both for minimizing your rosacea outbreaks and for managing them when they do occur.

Chapter 7 outlined the kinds of foods that serve your health and your skin. Here in this chapter we'll describe these foods in more detail, and we'll suggest a range of proportions for them, so you can get a sense of how to put your meals together, whether you are preparing them at home or eating out.

The Standard Choice: The Food Pyramid

You may have heard of the food pyramid, which is the latest dietary standard put forth by the USDA in an attempt to provide nutritional a guideline for everyone. The food pyramid is a visual diagram of food groups arranged in a pyramid-shaped stack to show the recommended proportion of your daily food intake that each group should represent. The food group at the bottom represents the largest proportion of your recommended food intake, while the group at the top represents the smallest proportion.

We believe there are some major problems with the food pyramid and its recommendations. As you can see by examining

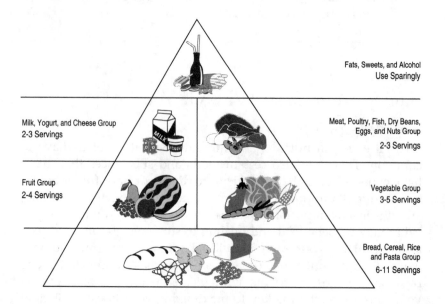

Fats, Sweets, and Alcohol
Use Sparingly

Milk, Yogurt, and Cheese Group
2-3 Servings

Meat, Poultry, Fish, Dry Beans, Eggs, and Nuts Group
2-3 Servings

Fruit Group
2-4 Servings

Vegetable Group
3-5 Servings

Bread, Cereal, Rice and Pasta Group
6-11 Servings

the food pyramid, the largest proportion of your recommended daily intake belongs to the "Bread, Cereal, Rice, and Pasta" group. This group is expected to represent about 60 to 70 percent of your total food intake per day.

Unfortunately, both processed grains and whole grains are lumped into the same recommended food group, with no distinction between the two. While whole grains, properly prepared, are nutritious and health supporting, there are a number of factors that make refined grains problematical. First, important nutrients are destroyed and discarded in the refining process. Second, many of these lost nutrients are critical for fully digesting and utilizing the carbohydrates that remain. This means that nutrient reserves already present in the body must be used to digest and absorb the carbohydrates, leading to possible nutrient depletion.

Furthermore, there is no distinction between the grains (and foods made from them) that are most commonly found to be problematic for some people, and those that are not. Many grains are a significant source of the digestive and food sensitivity problems that are so common today (Gottschall 1997). For example, wheat, and the gluten that is in the wheat and in many other grains, are a major source of food sensitivity (Lalles and Peltre 1996). As we mentioned in the previous chapters, the protein (gluten) in grains is one of the hardest proteins for humans to digest.

Finally, the recommendation does not address the fact that most grains contain phytates and enzyme inhibitors that can inhibit mineral absorption (Halberg 1987) and weaken you're your own intestinal enzymes, thereby inhibiting adequate digestion of foods made from these grains (Fallon and Enig 1999). Ways to prepare grains that will mitigate these problems are given later in this chapter.

Also, you'll notice that all dairy products are lumped together, with no distinction between cow, goat, and sheep dairy. But, just as with the grain-based food group, dairy products are not all the same. Cow dairy products are among the most common sources of both allergies and digestive problems, while goat dairy is often better tolerated (Krohn 1991). This may be true of sheep dairy as well. Also, the recommendations make no distinction as to how the milk is produced or processed. Raw milk from healthy, pasture-fed animals, containing its natural enzymes, is the ideal, and much more nourishing and easier to digest than most supermarket milk (Schmid 1987). Cultured foods, like yogurt and kefir, in which lactic acid-producing bacteria have already begun digesting both the milk protein and the milk sugar, are much more digestible than uncultured dairy.

Perhaps most problematic of all, especially for those with rosacea, is that fats and oils are allotted only the smallest portion of the food pyramid, as though all fats and oils are the same and are barely beneficial for you. Fats and oils, *the right fats and oils*, are not only beneficial for you in many ways, but are absolutely essential for healthy skin. This will be addressed in considerably more detail later on.

Our Recommendation: The Food Wheel

A good visual representation of the daily food intake we recommend would not be a food pyramid at all, but a *food wheel*. Look carefully at it. There is a sort of fluid and natural flow to the food wheel.

As you can see, at the center of the wheel is the vegetables food group, which functions as a kind of core around which the other food groups are arranged. The circles that surround this center represent protein foods of various kinds, protein/carbohydrate combination foods, fats and oils, fruits, and water. The food groups in the food wheel represent those foods that are nourishing and beneficial to most people. The sizes of the circles are approximate and will vary according to individual nutritional needs.

The dietary suggestions below may be very different from how you are used to eating. As you work toward eating these types of food, you may discover a new level of health. Change isn't always easy, and taking it gradually allows the process to become a natural part of our lives. Start slowly if that suits you, but make it a goal to eat healthier. Your skin should start improving and you may well find yourself feeling much better in general.

Vegetable Foods

About 60 to 65 percent of the entire quantity of food that you take in each day (representing 30 to 35 percent of calories) should consist of vegetables. They provide phytonutrients, antioxidants, soluble and insoluble fiber, as well as minerals and vitamins that complement other healthful components of your diet. One of the important benefits of fresh vegetables is that they help keep your body from becoming too acidic. The internal environment of your body is slightly alkaline, i.e., just above pH 7.0. If your tissues become too acidic, your body uses minerals like potassium, calcium, magnesium, and others to buffer the acids and excrete them. Over time, this can deplete the body of needed minerals and lead to a buildup of excess acids in your tissues, which can burden your immune system and keep it under a continuous state of distress. Excess acid waste in your body can stimulate a variety of problems, including chronic infections, digestive difficulties, and allergies. This can reduce the efficiency of energy production in the cells, leaving you more susceptible to fatigue, illness, and pain (Anderson, Rosenbaum, and Bland 1999). Since your skin is

FOOD WHEEL

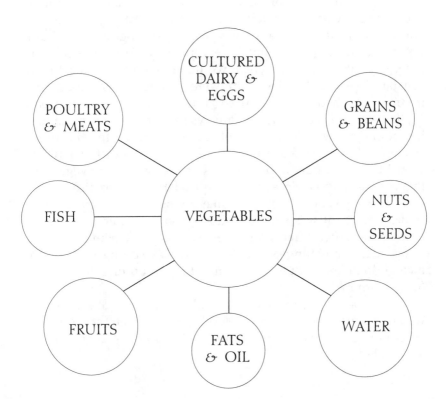

an eliminative organ, it would of course be affected. You can imagine the impact of this on your ability to manage your rosacea.

You may have heard of the acid/alkaline diet, which basically allows you to regulate the acidity or alkalinity of your body tissues by understanding which foods tend to generate more systemic acidity and which ones create more alkalinity. It seems that so many of our favorite foods, and particularly those we feel "addicted" to, are acid-forming. Vegetables, on the other hand, are our major alkalinizing foods, as are most fruits.

Eric, a construction worker near Indianapolis, found that his rosacea outbreaks were more prevalent in warm weather. Because the summers were usually hot and muggy, and his job was physically demanding, he expected this to be pretty much what he would have to put up with every year. Then an interesting thing happened. "A friend of mine turned me on to something he read in a health magazine about acid-forming and alkaline-forming foods. When I read about the foods that tend to make your system more acidic and the ones that make you more alkaline, something about it made sense—especially since most everything I was eating fell into the 'acid-forming' category. I got this weird feeling that maybe it was affecting my skin. I didn't really like vegetables much, except for corn on the cob and potatoes. But I figured maybe it would be worth a try to eat more vegetables, especially since they were in season right then. Plus, my neighbor had a huge garden and was always trying to pass off his vegetables anyway. He always grew five times more than he could eat. I wasn't comfortable cutting back on the size of my steaks so I could make room for the rabbit food, but I did it. Weird thing is, after about ten days of taking in more vegetables than I'd usually eat in a year, I noticed I wasn't as tired at the end of the day. And it seemed like my skin was doing better. I figured maybe it was wishful thinking, so I'd better give it some more time. After three more weeks, I stopped being afraid to think it. It *was* getting better. Maybe it was cutting back on the meat, I don't know. But I know this—I'm not putting down rabbit food anymore."

For your reference, we've included an Acid/Alkaline Chart, which shows where various foods fall on the acid/alkaline spectrum, in terms of the pH *after* the food is digested and assimilated.

Acid/Alkaline Chart

Most Alkaline	More Alkaline	Low Alkaline	Lowest Alkaline
Baking soda	Spices/cinnamon	Herbs (most)	Ginger tea
Sea salt	Soy sauce	Green tea	
	Molasses	Rice syrup	Sucanat
Pumpkin seed	Poppy seed	Apple cider vinegar	Umeboshi vinegar
		Sake	
Lentils	Cashews	Sesame seed	
Brocoflower	Chestnuts	Almonds	
Seaweeds	Pepper	Sprouts	Ghee (clarified butter)
Onion	Kohlrabi	Quail eggs	Duck eggs
Miso, soy sauce	Parsnip/taro	Primrose oil	Oats
Daikon/taro root	Garlic	Avocado	Quinoa
Burdock root	Asparagus	Potato/bell pepper	Wild rice
Sweet potato/ yam	Kale/parsley	Mushroom/fungi	Japonica rice
Lime	Endive/arugala	Cauliflower	Coconut oil
Nectarine	Mustard greens	Cabbage	Olive oil
Persimmon	Ginger root	Rutabaga	Flax oil
Raspberry	Broccoli	Eggplant	Brussel sprout
Watermelon	Grapefruit	Pumpkin	Beet
Tangerine	Cantaloupe	Collard greens	Chive/cilantro
Pineapple	Honeydew	Cod liver oil	Celery
Umeboshi plums	Citrus	Lemon	Okra/cucumber
	Olive	Papaya	Turnip greens
	Loganberry	Pear	Squashes
	Mango	Apple	Lettuces
		Blackberry	Jicama
		Cherry	Orange
		Peach	Apricot
			Banana
			Blueberry
			Strawberry
			Grape
			Raisin/currant

Lowest Acid	Low Acid	More Acid	Most Acid
Honey/maple syrup	Stevia	Aspartame	Sugar
Curry	Vanilla	Coffee	Table salt
Kona coffee	Black tea	Butter (chocolate)	Cocoa
Cream/butter	Goat milk	Milk protein	Pudding/ jam/jelly
Goat/sheep cheeses		Cottage cheese	Yeast/hops/ malt
Yogurt	Aged cheese	New cheeses	Beer
Chicken eggs	Soy cheese	Soy milk	Processed cheese
Rice vinegar	Balsamic vinegar		White/acetic vinegar
Gelatin/organ meats	Lamb/mutton	Pork/veal	Ice cream
Venison	Boar/elk	Bear	Soy
Wild duck	Goose/turkey	Chicken	Beef
Fish	Shellfish/mollusks	Mussels/squid	Lobster
		Lard	Pheasant
Triticale	Buckwheat	Maize	Barley
Millet	Wheat	Corn	Cottonseed oil/meal
Kasha (buckwheat)	Spelt/teff/kamut	Rye	Hazelnuts
Amaranth	Farina/seminola	Oat bran	Walnuts
Brown rice	White rice	Pecans	Fried foods
Pine nuts	Seitan	Pistachio seed	Carob
Grape seed oil	Tapioca	Peanut	
Sunflower oil	Safflower oil	Chick pea/garbanzo	
Pumpkin seed oil	Almond oil	Snow pea	
Canola oil	Sesame oil	Carrots	
Fava beans	Tofu	Palm kernel oil	
Kidney beans	Pinto beans	Green pea	
Black-eyed beans	White beans	Cranberry	
String/wax beans	Navy/red beans	Pomegranate	
	Aduki beans		
	Lima beans		
Spinach	Chard		
Coconut	Plum/prune		
Guava	Tomatoes		
Figs			
Dates			
Dry fruit			

Chart courtesy Serammune Physician's Lab, 14 Pigeon Hill Drive #300, Sterling, VA 20165

Nonstarchy Vegetables

These foods are particularly important. Examples are broccoli, green beans, snap peas (including the edible pod), snow peas, artichokes, chicory, collards, chard, dandelion greens, garlic, kale (all kinds), zucchini, summer squash, kohlrabi, celery, cucumbers, bok choy, zucchini, leeks, scallions, onions, baby mixed lettuces, spinach, dark leafy greens (especially Romaine lettuce), parsley, radicchio, and radishes. These vegetables, especially if they are grown organically and lightly cooked, provide the B vitamin folic acid. Folic acid is particularly important because it works in partnership with vitamin B_{12} to support the immune system and nourish the skin. These vegetables also provide wonderful antioxidants for your skin such as lycopene and beta carotene.

Starchy Vegetables

These are also important to include in your diet. These include root vegetables such as rutabagas, turnips, parsnips, beets (red, orange, yellow), potatoes, sweet potatoes, yams, carrots, and gourd-type vegetables such as all the winter squashes and, of course, pumpkins. These also contain carotenes (beta, alpha, etc.) and valuable minerals, especially when grown in rich soil.

Protein Foods

Unless you are engaged in heavy exercise or muscle-building, your daily intake of protein should be limited to about 25 to 30 percent of your caloric intake. There are many foods to choose from, depending on what appeals to you.

Animal Protein Foods

About 15 to 20 percent of your food intake each day can consist of healthy animal protein foods, which also contain healthy natural fats. These foods also contain B vitamins, including B_{12} and biotin, both highly valuable for the immune system and the skin. The B's are needed for mental/emotional well-being as well. These foods also contain vitamins A and D, both of which have been used for inflammatory conditions of the skin. They also contain minerals if the food supply of the livestock was rich in minerals. The foods that fall into this category are:

Fresh fish (*not shellfish*, however, since they may unfortunately harbor high levels of contaminants). Examples are salmon, ahi tuna, red snapper, rainbow trout, cod, mackerel, pickerel, whitefish, sea trout, carp, monkfish, yellow perch, silver perch, albacore tuna, mahi-mahi, ocean perch, pike, sea bass, sturgeon, shark, swordfish, yellowtail, and white perch.

Poultry—organic or at least hormone/antibiotic-free if possible. This includes chicken, turkey, and game birds.

Cultured dairy products such as plain goat yogurt, goat cheeses, or, if well tolerated, cultured cow's milk products such as plain yogurt, kefir, and various cheeses. Organic raw milk products that have been cultured are great if you can find them. There are two different problems that some people have with dairy products: allergy and lactose intolerance. Dairy allergy involves a reaction to casein and/or other proteins in the milk; people with these allergies must avoid dairy products. Lactose intolerance, however, is a deficiency in the enzyme lactase, which is necessary for digesting the lactose found in uncultured dairy products. If dairy causes stomach pains, bloating, and gas, you are probably in this category. There are supplements that you can take that will supply the lactase enzyme you need so that you can enjoy these foods in your diet.

Beef and lamb (organic or at least hormone/antibiotic-free if possible) in moderation.

Vegetable Protein Foods

Another source of protein in your diet is vegetable protein/carbohydrate combination foods. About 10 to 15 percent of your caloric intake each day can consist of vegetable protein foods, which also contain lots of natural carbohydrate. These foods contain B vitamins like B_2 and B_6, as well as minerals. The foods that fall into this category are:

Grains and beans: These are the protein-rich foods of the vegetable world. They contain valuable nutrients, but they also contain phytates and enzyme-inhibiting factors that can make these foods very difficult to digest. If you aren't able to digest them thoroughly, they can end up irritating your intestinal lining. This can lead to a condition called intestinal permeability, or "leaky gut," which is believed to play a role in many inflammatory conditions. (See chapter 9 for how this might relate to rosacea for some people.) To destroy a good portion of their phytate and anti-enzyme content and make them more easily digestible, you can culture or sprout grains and beans before cooking. Traditional cultures all over the world have used both of these methods for millennia. Follow these steps to culture organic whole grains (preferably oats, barley, millet, amaranth, red/black/brown rices), dried organic whole beans, or canned and *drained* black, pinto, navy, soy, red, or any other preferred beans):

- ※ Determine how much you want to cook and set aside. (You can grind or crush grains fresh, which helps them to culture even more thoroughly, and then set them aside.)

- ※ *Using the pan you will be cooking the grains or beans in,* fill it with enough lukewarm water to provide a 3:1 ratio of water to grains.

- ※ Add 1 to 2 tablespoons organic plain yogurt, either goat or cow (or use 2 or more caps of a probiotic), or natural whey, or even lemon juice.

- ※ Stir yogurt (or probiotic, whey, or lemon juice)/water mixture until all is thoroughly dissolved and dispersed.

- ※ Add in the grains or beans (dried, or canned and drained) and stir well.

- ※ Cover and set aside at room temperature for 24 hours (only 7 hours needed for rice, although longer is even better).

- ※ After 24 hours (or longer if desired), follow these steps:

For grains: Keep the grains in the soaking liquid and place the pan on the stove. Add a large pinch of Celtic sea salt (which should be available at most good health food grocers) and cook slowly for 1 hour (it may take less because of the soaking and culturing, or it may take more if you are cooking a large amount of grains).

For dried beans: Drain the soaking water off, rinse beans, and place back in pot. Add enough water to cover the beans. Add a large pinch of Celtic sea salt and bring to a boil for several minutes, skimming off foam. Add garlic and/or other herbs/spices as desired. Reduce heat and simmer, covered, for 4 to 8 hours.

For canned beans: Keep the beans in the soaking water; add a large pinch of Celtic sea salt. Bring to a boil for several minutes, skimming off any foam (there may be very little or none). Add garlic and or other herbs and spices as desired. Reduce heat and simmer, covered, for 1 to 2 hours.

Cultured hot grains are great for breakfast served with organic cultured butter or a dollop of organic yogurt. Top with freshly ground flaxseed meal. You can cook up large amounts of grains or beans and then when they've cooled down, divide them up into containers and freeze for future meals. To use, just pull out a frozen container and leave it at room temperature for 7 to 8 hours or overnight. Transfer to a stovetop pan for a quick heat-up.

If you prefer your grains in the form of breads, try to find a bread that is made from sprouted grains (no flour). Another possibility is to find a bread that is made from flour that has been freshly ground and immediately subjected to a special, very slow, cool fermentation process, which significantly reduces the phytate and enzyme-inhibiting factors in the grains.

Nuts: Nuts are best used sparingly, because they also contain enzyme-inhibiting factors. Also, many people are fairly sensitive to nuts, and some even have allergic reactions to them, as noted in chapter 7. The digestibility of nuts can be enhanced by soaking them overnight, then drying them slowly in a lukewarm oven and storing them in an airtight container (Fallon and Enig 1999).

Fruits

About 10 to 15 percent of your caloric intake each day should consist of fresh fruits. Fruits are natural carbohydrate foods that are rich in antioxidants and minerals, such as vitamin C and hundreds of bioflavonoids including proanthocyanidins, anthocyanidins, catechins, hesperidin, rutin, and many more, all of which promote good immune function and help strengthen capillaries. Fruits also provide many minerals, which are essential for healing tissue. Fruits fall into two categories:

Acid and Sub-acid Fruits

Examples of this type of fruit are plums, figs, black cherries, apples, pears, Asian pears, peaches, nectarines, apricots, blueberries, elderberries, raspberries, blackberries, cranberries, cherries, grapes, pineapple, kiwi, pomegranates, Fuyu persimmons, and citrus fruits if tolerated.

Sweet and Starchy Fruits

Examples are all melons, mangoes, papayas, bananas, and soft persimmons. These fruits have a higher sugar content than the acid and sub-acid fruits.

Fats and Oils

About 25 to 30 percent of your caloric intake each day should consist of a healthy balance of fats and oils, all of which are known in the nutritional biochemistry world as *fatty acids*. The fatty acids that will serve you well fall into the following categories:

Sources of Omega-3, Omega-6, and Omega-9 Fatty Acids

Olive oil to provide monounsaturated omega-9 fatty acid.

EPA and DHA fish body oil to provide two special omega-3 fatty acids, EPA and DHA. EPA helps keep inflammatory conditions under control. DHA is particularly important for neurological and brain health. EPA and DHA are found in fish, especially raw or rare fish, as well as in fish oil capsules.

Cod liver oil to provide truly natural vitamin A and vitamin D, as well as moderate amounts of EPA and DHA omega-3 fatty acids. It is critical to get carefully selected, meticulously processed fish oil in antioxidant-protected capsules.

Borage oil to provide a special omega-6 fatty acid called GLA (gamma linolenic acid), a special form of omega-6 fatty acid. You can obtain this either in liquid or capsule form. You can also use capsules of evening primrose oil or black currant oil, both of which contain GLA, although in lesser amounts.

Whole avocado (not the extracted oil). Avocado is one of the few sources of natural, unadulterated, unprocessed omega-6 and omega-9 fatty acids.

Sesame oil (*non-toasted* only); provides omega-6 fatty acids, and contains sesamin, reported to reduce hypertension (Gaby 1997). Use in moderation, since you don't want to overload with too much omega-6.

Flax oil in small amounts only, up to one tablespoon a day, to provide the plant-based (ALA) form of omega-3 fatty acid. This oil cannot tolerate heat, so do not use it for cooking. You can also use flaxmeal as a source of this oil. Try a couple of tablespoons sprinkled on any foods you like. It's great on yogurt, cereal, or your favorite vegetables.

Important information about omega-3 oils:

❀ Keep all your omega-3 oils in the freezer (the freezer door is a great place). The oils are highly susceptible to damaging oxidation, and an extremely cold storage temperature helps protect them from this. They will remain liquid, unless your freezer is extremely cold. If you are using flaxmeal, be sure to keep it in the freezer as well, since grinding up the seed exposes some of the oil to oxygen (although it's less exposed than when in the oil form).

❀ Keep your omega-3 oils away from heat. Although cooking fish isn't a problem, the extracted fish oils are very fragile and easily damaged by heat, so omega-3 oils should never be used for cooking. They are also easily damaged by light and are therefore provided in dark bottles that block light.

❀ Be sure to take vitamin E, in the natural mixed tocopherol form, along with your polyunsaturated oils like the omega-3 oils (flax oil or fish oils [including cod liver oil]). These oils are extremely sensitive to damage from oxidation, and the Vitamin E protects against this. Other antioxidants such as Vitamin C, bioflavonoids, carotenoids, and proanthocyanadins can also help (Schmidt 1997). The best natural sources for these, of course, are fresh vegetables and fruits, but they are also available in supplement form.

Saturated Fats:

Naturally occurring animal fats (organic, or at least hormone/antibiotic-free if possible). Examples are butter, especially cultured butter, and other dairy products rich in beneficial short-chain and medium-chain saturated fatty acids, such as butyric acid, lauric acid, capric acid, caprylic acid, conjugated linoleic acid, as well as glycolipids (Enig 2000). These fats are found naturally in the body fat of clean fish, organically raised, grass-fed sheep and beef, and free-running poultry, as well as in the egg yolks from this poultry. Butter also contains natural vitamin A and D, especially if the animals are grass-fed (Fallon and Enig 1999). (Animal fats also contain unsaturated fatty acids.)

Ghee (clarified butter) is butter that has had all the milk solids removed, leaving only the butterfat. It's wonderful for light sautéing because it has a higher heat tolerance than oils. Contains butyric acid.

Coconut oil is also great for light cooking because of its high heat tolerance; it contains lauric acid.

Why Are the Right Fats and Oils So Important?

Well, let's think about this: Each cell of your body is contained within a membrane, kind of like a water balloon, and many of the functional units inside each cell are contained within their own membranes as well. Fatty acids are a major component of these membranes.

To make healthy cell membranes, your body must have healthy, appropriately balanced fatty acids. This means that *the quality of the membranes of every cell of every tissue in your body is dependent on the kinds of fatty acids* that you consume. Healthy cell membranes structurally support your cells, get adequate oxygen into them, help them to generate energy, respond correctly to hormonal signals, eliminate waste, and allow the cells to replicate as healthy cells rather than cancer cells. This affects all the tissues of your body—your skin and connective tissue, brain and nerve tissue, muscle tissue, bones, all your internal organs, your red blood cells, your white blood cells, even your hair follicle cells!

Whatever fatty acids you take in through your foods, your body will use. For example, if you take in trans fatty acids, they will end up in your body's tissues and have an effect on the way the organs in your body function. Your system will use these "bad" fatty acids to make new cell membranes, which will not have the strength and integrity of healthy cell membranes (Enig 2000, Schmidt 1997). If you think of this in terms of the cells of your skin and connective tissues, it means that the health of these tissues requires a consistent and plentiful supply of the right fats and oils.

Some Considerations Regarding Fats

✳ Although you might be wary of them, the truth is that your body needs natural saturated fats. According to Dr. Mary Enig, an internationally known lipid biochemist and nutritionist, in her new book *Know Your Fats*, the body needs saturated fats for at least half of the fatty acid part of the phospholipids that form cell membranes. She notes that research has shown that saturated fat in the diet is needed by the body to enable it to adequately convert the essential omega-3 fatty acid (alpha-linolenic acid) to the EPA and DHA omega-3 fatty acids. In fact, the human body will even *make* saturated fats because it requires them. Animal fats are actually a natural mixture of saturated and unsaturated fatty acids, often with the larger percentage of the mix being *unsaturated*.

✳ Healthy, naturally occurring animal and dairy fats provide a number of highly valuable and unique *saturated* fatty acids. Because of their health benefits for the intestinal lining, they can be very helpful in reducing inflammation.

✳ These same natural animal and dairy fats provide some valuable *unsaturated* fatty acids that are not found in other foods.

✳ These fats have been a significant part of the diets of healthy human cultures all over the world for millennia—cultures that have been known for longevity and that have existed for centuries free from today's degenerative diseases. In fact, these fats were recognized and venerated by these traditional cultures as essential for a strong, viable, disease-free community (Fallon and Enig 1999).

Over the past several decades, we've seen a large portion of these natural fats shoved aside by the influx of hydrogenated and partially hydrogenated fats and oils and the products made from them that are the major source of trans fatty acids in our diet today. Many of us in the United States still do use plenty of animal and dairy fats. Unfortunately, what is currently most available to us are products of conventional agricultural methods. This means we are faced with taking in residues of pesticides, herbicides, fungicides, antibiotics, and growth hormones along with what should be healthy, nourishing foods. What to do? Do whatever you can to acquire your animal and dairy products from organic sources, or "clean" sources that provide them as free from chemical residue as possible. If you can't find a clean source, then it's still important to include these animal and dairy fat sources. It may be a question of trial and error, since it's possible for the chemicals that end up in these conventional foods to affect your immune system and contribute to your rosacea problem.

❋ Your body also needs healthy sources of cholesterol for healthy cell membranes and tissue repair, including connective tissue and skin, for nerve health, and for healthy hormonal balance through life (Enig 2000). Taking in some natural cholesterol through the diet provides some relief to your liver, which is responsible for making whatever cholesterol the body requires beyond that which comes in through the diet. According to Dr. Enig, "The evidence is clear that for most people the more that dietary cholesterol is ingested, the less it is synthesized by their body tissues" (57). Also, she notes that high serum cholesterol *decreases* with consumption of most fatty acids, including all saturates.

❋ Omega-3, omega-6, and omega-9 fatty acids are critically important. In fact, the omega-3 fatty acid alpha-linoleic acid and the omega-6 fatty acid linoleic acid are called *essential fatty acids*, because they are the only ones that cannot be made in the body and must be supplied through the diet. It has been recently found that in Western industrialized society, far more of the omega-6 oils are taken in, perhaps too much, and not enough of the omega-3s (Crayhon 1994). Studies have indicated that omega-3 deficiency is associated with allergies and inflammatory conditions (Clinical Pearls 1997). Correcting these deficiencies has been therapeutic for psoriasis, eczema, asthma, lupus, high blood pressure, high serum cholesterol levels, and even cancer (Nouochi 1995; DeVries and Van Noorden 1992). We feel that a ratio of about 1:1.5:2 of omega-3: omega-6: omega-9 is optimal.

❋ Avoid the wrong kinds of fatty acids, including: overheated oils, oxidized fats/oils, hydrogenated or partially hydrogenated oils, and trans fatty acids (where the oil molecule is twisted due to over-processing or overheating). In addition to their harm to cell membranes, these trans fats may be used by your body to make other fatty acids that are not health promoting.

❋ Avoid, *if you can*, fats that come from conventionally raised animals, which may have absorbed residues from pesticides, herbicides, fungicides, hormones, and possibly other chemicals from conventional farming and processing practices. You might even check the Web for good sources. But don't despair if you only have conventional sources available—your body will still enjoy the fatty acids they contain.

How Fatty Acids Can Affect Inflammatory Conditions

Since some of the beneficial fats and oils that we've listed may not be that familiar to you, here is some additional information about them that may be helpful. If this is more information on fats than you really care to know, you can skip this part and just use the recommendations for fats and oils given in chapter 7. For those who are interested in reading more about fatty acids, the following information might be helpful in understanding the role they can play in regulating inflammatory responses in your body. Given that rosacea involves inflammation, you may find this information to be very useful in terms of possibly managing your rosacea.

Omega-6 and omega-3 fatty acids play a key role in regulating inflammatory processes in your body by their transformation into substances called *prostaglandins*, also called *eicosanoids*.

Fatty Acid Chart

Key: **SF:** <u>Saturated Fat</u> (naturally saturated fatty acid)

AA: <u>Arachidonic Acid</u> (a form of Omega-6 fatty acid that occurs in <u>grain-fed</u> animal fat and egg yolks)

GLA: <u>Gamma Linolenic Acid</u> (a derivative of Omega-6 fatty acids)

EPA/DHA: <u>Eicosapentaenoic Acid</u>/<u>Docosahexaenoic Acid</u> (two special Omega-3's that occur in fish and seaweed)

Ω6: Omega-6 fatty acid (a polyunsaturated fatty acid)

Ω3: Omega-3 fatty acid (also a polyunsaturated fatty acid)

Ω9: Omega-9 fatty acid (a monounsaturated fatty acid)

PGE 1, 2, 3: Prostaglandins 1, 2, & 3; powerful hormone-like molecules that regulate cellular function

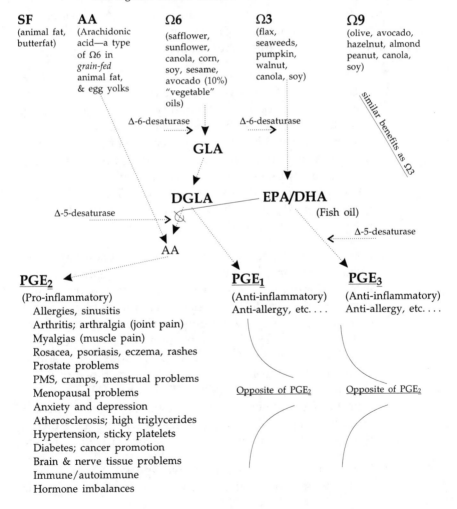

SF
(animal fat, butterfat)

AA
(Arachidonic acid—a type of Ω6 in *grain-fed* animal fat, & egg yolks)

Ω6
(safflower, sunflower, canola, corn, soy, sesame, avocado (10%) "vegetable" oils)

Ω3
(flax, seaweeds, pumpkin, walnut, canola, soy)

Ω9
(olive, avocado, hazelnut, almond peanut, canola, soy)

similar benefits as Ω3

Δ-6-desaturase

Δ-6-desaturase

GLA

DGLA — **EPA/DHA**
(Fish oil)

Δ-5-desaturase

Δ-5-desaturase

AA

PGE$_2$

(Pro-inflammatory)
Allergies, sinusitis
Arthritis; arthralgia (joint pain)
Myalgias (muscle pain)
Rosacea, psoriasis, eczema, rashes
Prostate problems
PMS, cramps, menstrual problems
Menopausal problems
Anxiety and depression
Atherosclerosis; high triglycerides
Hypertension, sticky platelets
Diabetes; cancer promotion
Brain & nerve tissue problems
Immune/autoimmune
Hormone imbalances

PGE$_1$

(Anti-inflammatory)
Anti-allergy, etc. . . .

<u>Opposite of PGE$_2$</u>

PGE$_3$

(Anti-inflammatory)
Anti-allergy, etc. . . .

<u>Opposite of PGE$_2$</u>

These prostaglandins are important hormone-like molecules that are created in all cells of your body. They have a powerful effect on the functioning of your cells, as well as a direct influence on your immune system. They are classified into three basic groups: PGE_2 (prostaglandin E_2), PGE_1 (prostaglandin E_1), and PGE_3 (prostaglandin E_3). PGE_2 is pro-inflammatory, while PGE_1 and PGE_3 are anti-inflammatory.

A few pages back, included in the list of fatty acids (fats and oils) that will serve you well, were borage oil, EPA and DHA fish body oil, and flax oil. Borage oil is in the omega-6 family, while fish body oil and flax oil are in the omega-3 family. There are important derivatives of these oils that work in a kind of partnership to help regulate the production of both the pro-inflammatory and anti-inflammatory eicosanoids, and thus offer considerable control over the inflammatory process in your body. The following might help explain this a little more:

- Borage oil is a source of GLA (gamma linolenic acid), a special form of omega-6 fatty acid that is essential for humans. Your body has the ability to manufacture GLA from the omega-6 oils in your diet, but for a number of reasons, your production of GLA can be limited, so it can be very helpful to get it through the diet. Borage oil is the most abundant source of already naturally formed GLA. GLA is transformed in your body to DGLA, which then gets converted into both the *anti*-inflammatory PGE_1 and the *pro*-inflammatory PGE_2.

- Flax oil and flaxmeal are probably the best sources of the plant-based omega-3 fatty acid ALA (alpha-linolenic acid). When you take in ALA, your body has the ability to convert it (through a series of steps) to the two special omega-3 fatty acids mentioned earlier, EPA and DHA. But if your health is less than optimal, this capacity can be relatively limited (Gerster 1998). If your body is able to make EPA, the EPA then gets further transformed to the anti-inflammatory PGE_3. There have been many reports of people enjoying considerable improvement in various inflammatory conditions by taking flax oil or flaxmeal (which naturally contains flax oil).

- Fish body oil is a source of two special omega-3 fatty acids, EPA, and DHA. These two fatty acids occur naturally and in good quantity in fish (especially wild fish), and in marine animals, as well as in wild meat and fowl. Since the body's capacity to make EPA and DHA from ALA can be limited, especially if your health is at all compromised, eating fresh fish and/or taking fish body oil is a great way to get EPA and DHA directly.

✳ With the help of a special enzyme (delta-5-desaturase), EPA is converted to the anti-inflammatory PGE_3. Interestingly enough, this same enzyme (delta-5-desaturase) is also required to convert DGLA to the pro-inflammatory PGE_2. When the EPA portion of fish oil is present, it "steals" much of the delta-5-desaturase enzyme from the PGE_2 pathway to use it for converting EPA to PGE_3, leaving less for conversion of DGLA to PGE_2. So you have a kind of competitive inhibition, which limits the amount of PGE_2 produced. (Take a look at the Fatty Acid Chart above to get a visual impression of this.) This has the effect of preventing the overproduction of PGE_2 and limiting it pro-inflammatory effects.

✳ An additional benefit of this is that as more of the enzyme is pulled away from the PGE_2 pathway, more of the DGLA conversion is directed toward production of the beneficial anti-inflammatory prostaglandin E_1 (PGE_1). The overall effect is an increase in both PGE_1 and PGE_3, and a decrease in PGE_2. The body can balance the pro- and anti-inflammatory effects as it requires.

A fatty acid success story: It's wonderful to hear stories about what people have tried as they've addressed the seemingly endless struggle to prevent rosacea outbreaks, or to at least put a quick end to them once they've begun. For example, George, a real estate salesman in Santa Fe, had recurring flare-ups, and nothing he tried seemed to help. He even attempted a macrobiotic diet for about a month. Then one day a friend of his found some information on the Web about flax oil and how people were reporting that it helped with different kinds of inflammation. He told George about it and George figured it was worth a try, so he ordered some. He took one tablespoon a day for about two weeks, and for the first time in several years, it seemed like something was finally working. His skin seemed less irritated and generally smoother. After about two months, he was elated to find that his outbreaks were less intense and they seemed to quiet down faster.

Here's a sample protocol you might want to try:

✳ Take 1 to 1½ teaspoons *fresh* (look for a recent pressing date on the bottle) organic flax oil twice a day, with your morning and evening meals; if you don't want to use the oil directly, you might want to try grinding up flax seeds to make fresh flaxmeal (in some places you may be able to find vacuum-packed, pre-ground flaxmeal). Use a teaspoon to a tablespoon (or more, if you like). Keep your flaxmeal in the freezer just like you do the flax oil.

✳ Take 2 gelcaps of borage oil twice a day with your morning and evening meals, or ½ to 1 teaspoon liquid borage oil twice a day with these meals.

✳ Also take vitamin E, 400 IU in natural mixed tocopherol form with your breakfast meal.

Some people find the fish oil (EPA and DHA) works better for them, so you may prefer to substitute fish oil gelcaps in place of the flax oil, enough to provide about 320 to 640 mg of EPA twice a day at meals. (If you intend to take more, you might want to check with a health care provider who is familiar with the benefits of essential fatty acids).

Essential fatty acids for ocular rosacea: Dry eye syndrome seems to be a fairly common problem with rosacea. It can be painful and frustrating. Fortunately, in some cases it has been found to respond very well to essential fatty acids. A case history might illustrate this.

Loretta, a twenty-six-year-old grad student, has spent most of her college days in front of a computer. A couple of years ago, she started having trouble with her eyes. They seemed red a lot of the time, and felt increasingly irritated. She tried regular eye drops, which actually seemed to make them worse. Her primary doctor gave her prescription eye drops, which seemed to make her vision blurry and gave her only temporary relief. Finally, she went to an ophthalmologist, who looked at her eyes, listened to her symptoms, and then diagnosed her with mild ocular rosacea.

Since her teens, Loretta had always felt the need to use a lot of lotion because her skin was so dry. She thought drinking ten glasses of water a day might help. But it was annoying to always need to be near a bathroom, and besides, having to get up several times a night was disturbing her sleep and leaving her feeling tired in the morning. And the bottom line was that all this water, by itself, wasn't helping either her dry skin or her eyes.

Loretta went to a nutritionist, and a review of her dietary intake revealed that she was taking in very little oil or fat, in an attempt to eat healthfully and keep her weight down. She wasn't suffering from any particular health problems, and had no history of difficulty in digesting fats and oils.

Although she was hesitant to introduce fats or oils into her diet, Loretta decided she might be willing to consider it when their role, particularly the role of omega-6 and omega-3 fatty acids, was explained to her. It seemed wise to start slowly since her system wasn't used to digesting fats or oils. She decided to use the flaxmeal rather than the flax oil, and she agreed to eat avocado, which she loved but had been avoiding as a fatty food. She also agreed to take borage oil capsules for their GLA content. Loretta's protocol looked like this:

Week 1:   1 teaspoon of flaxmeal with breakfast +
           1 teaspoon with dinner.
        Half an avocado at lunch.
        1 borage oil capsule (300 mg) at dinner.

Week 2:   2 teaspoons of flaxmeal with breakfast +
           2 teaspoons with dinner.
        Half an avocado at lunch.
        1 borage oil capsule (300 mg) at breakfast +
           1 at dinner.

Week 3:   1 tablespoon of flaxmeal with breakfast + 1 table
           spoon at dinner.
        Half an avocado at lunch.
        1 borage oil capsule (300 mg) at breakfast +
           1 at dinner.

At the end of the third week, she reported that her eyes felt less gritty but were still irritated. She was then advised to increase her intake of fish (she chose lightly cooked salmon). Loretta continued this regimen for another two months, and then checked back in. By this time she had stopped using any eye drops. She said eyes were hardly bothering her at all now, and they certainly looked much better. As an added benefit, the skin on her whole body had become far less dry.

As you can see, there is a lot of information about the kinds of foods and drink that will truly nourish your body and give it the proper nutrients that it needs to restore and maintain healthy skin. In chapter 7, you learned that, on average, you take in about a ton of food and drink per year. In fact, there may be no way that you are in more intimate contact with your environment, on a consistent and repetitive basis, than by way of what you eat and drink every day. It stands to reason that the impact of this is no less than profound. That's why we believe that addressing your nutritional intake is at the core of a well-rounded process that can help you successfully manage your rosacea.

9

How You Eat

Is it really necessary to talk about that unglamorous process—digestion? As unappealing as it may seem, an understanding of what happens *after* you swallow your food is essential for seeing how the digestive process can profoundly affect what's going on with your skin.

Saving Your Face ... HOW You Eat and Drink

To give you a sense of what your digestion is really about, let's focus on three major kinds of foods that demonstrate the three fundamental ways that your digestive system processes your foods: *fruits, starches,* and *proteins.* As you continue, it will become clearer why these foods have been selected for discussion. If you want a deeper explanation of the digestive process, take a look at the section later in this chapter called "Protectors and Enemies in Your Gut."

Fruit Digestion

Fruits are probably the easiest and quickest to digest of all your natural foods. For the sake of understanding, assume you take in some fruit on an empty stomach. You chew it up fairly quickly and swallow it down. It requires very little activity in your stomach, and within thirty to forty-five minutes it has passed on to your intestines, where within an hour or even less the digestion of it is complete. The total time is somewhere around ninety minutes.

Starch Digestion

By starches, we're referring to all the carbohydrate foods that are made primarily from grains: wheat, rye, oats, barley, corn, rice, etc. Again, assuming your stomach is empty, let's say you eat some starch in the form of a piece of bread. Starch requires more chewing than fruit, so it takes longer. Then it passes into your stomach, where it lingers longer than fruit—perhaps an hour or more—in order to break down the small amount of protein that might be present in the bread. Then it passes into your small intestine, where the digestive process is completed as the starch is broken down into glucose. The total time for all this may be two and a half to four hours.

Protein Digestion

Proteins are a different story. In order to best explain protein digestion, we'll focus mainly on the very concentrated animal proteins (fish, poultry, meat, egg, dairy). The chewing time required for these proteins is considerably longer (although they are often not chewed thoroughly enough) than for starches or fruits. Next the protein passes into your stomach, which has the ability to detect the concentrated protein. Your stomach then goes into action, secreting a strong concentration of HCL (hydrochloric acid). This HCL basically sterilizes your food: some call it our first line of defense against disease-causing microbes. This HCL also triggers your stomach to produce large quantities of protein-digesting enzymes, which break down the protein from large protein molecules into chains of molecules known as polypeptides. This is Stage 1 of protein digestion, and it is a critical step.

The polypeptides from Stage 1 are then passed into your small intestine, where specialized protease (protein digesting) enzymes are designed to break them down into smaller peptides and amino acids (Stage 2 of protein digestion). These enzymes are programmed to work on polypeptides, rather than whole proteins.

If your HCL production is compromised, either because not enough of it is produced, or it gets diluted or diffused—whatever the reason—your stomach walls may not produce an adequate supply of enzymes to break down the protein into polypeptides. This means that Stage 1 doesn't get completed fully, and whole protein molecules can end up passing into your small intestine. When this happens, the enzymes in your small intestine are unable to complete the protein digestion process, and this undigested protein then becomes a food source for the undesirable bacteria there.

Unfortunately, the problem of compromised HCL production and the resulting insufficiency of protein-digesting enzymes increases with age, and the consequences of this are profound (Lipski 2000). A number of sources list rosacea as a symptom or condition associated with hypochlorhydria (low stomach acid). There are several factors that can contribute to this situation, some of which may already be familiar to you:

- Protein foods are often not thoroughly chewed.

- Protein foods are combined with other foods that don't require much (if any) HCL or protein digesting enzymes.

- Too much liquid is taken in with your meal—especially liquid that is acidic and/or carbonated, such as alcohol, coffee (highly acidic), beer, soda, mineral water, etc.

- The food is full of overheated/oxidized oils and fats.

- Sugars (often in hidden form) are included.

- Your daily eating pattern consists of "starvation" followed by overeating.

Tips for Improving Protein Digestion

We'll take these points one by one so you can really see how important they are. As you read on, it should become a little more clear how the different requirements for digestion of fruits, starches, and proteins affect your ability to digest them well. Here are some suggestions you can try for yourself.

Chew thoroughly. This assures that your food is physically broken down into fine particles, maximizing its surface area so that the HCL and enzymes in your stomach can thoroughly penetrate it and properly break it down for delivery to your small intestine. Chewing thoroughly also provides maximum opportunity for a special immunoglobulin substance in your saliva (called secretory IgA) to thoroughly penetrate each mouthful of food and inhibit the overgrowth of pathogens that are always present in foods. This helps protect the beneficial flora that live in your intestines and eases the load on the lymph tissue that resides in your intestinal walls.

Try eating the protein part of your meal first, to whatever extent is possible. In other words, rather than starting your meal with breads or other foods, actually start with the protein part of your meal (fish, poultry, meat, etc.). This is an adaptation of food combining principles, which originated literally a century ago with the Hay system. The idea is that the presence of nonprotein foods (starches, fruits, etc.) that don't require HCL can signal the stomach to produce less HCL, which, in turn, can limit the production of your protein-digesting enzymes. Although few studies have been done to support this claim, one study done in 1936 and reported in *Food Combining for Health* (1987), by Doris Grant and Jean Joice, demonstrated that HCL production, although high one and a quarter hours after protein was consumed by itself, was compromised when protein was consumed along with starch. Also, after the combined meal, proteins were digested with difficulty. In addition, it may be that the nonprotein foods, particularly starches, can absorb some of the HCL, making it less available for the protein foods that actually need it.

However, since HCL production and initial protein digestion occur primarily in the lower part of the stomach, it has been theorized that proteins and starches may be consumed in the same meal if the protein portion is taken first. Following this practice alone, many people have reported remarkable improvements in their digestion, and some health care providers have begun to recommend it (Golan 1995).

It may help to think of the letters **P-V-S**, meaning that you start your meal by eating the majority of the **P**rotein portion before engaging in the rest of your meal. Follow the protein with nonstarchy **V**egetables, either lightly cooked or a combination of lightly cooked and raw. Then, as you complete the majority of the vegetable portion of your meal, you can finish up with the **S**tarch foods, such as starchy vegetables, rice, pastas, breads, etc. If the protein part of your meal is vegetarian protein, which would be some kind of bean and grain combination (for example, tofu and long grain brown rice), then this becomes the protein portion of your meal, because it would contain more protein than the rest of your meal. (Although when eaten as part of a meal containing animal protein, the rice or other grain can be considered a "starch," in this case it can be considered the protein portion of your meal.)

Following the P-V-S pattern of food intake at a meal can provide an excellent chance of thoroughly digesting your food rather than have it feed harmful microorganisms in your intestines. Experiment with it and see if you notice any difference in your digestion and even in your overall well-being.

Minimize liquids at meals. Too much liquid with your meal can either dilute your HCL or—in the case of carbonated liquids—even neutralize it. Neutralizing your HCL can, in turn, inhibit the production and effectiveness of your protein-digestion enzymes. However, a small amount of liquid, such as a small glass of water or wine, sipped throughout the meal is not a problem.

Exclude overheated/oxidized or hydrogenated oils and fats. These fats and oils can interfere with the cellular energy required for enzyme production and thereby weaken digestion and absorption (Kunin 1999). Also, they contribute to the formation of unhealthy cell membranes (see chapter 8). However, *light* sautéing (which does not involve overheating) using olive oil, organic ghee, or even organic coconut oil is fine.

Eliminate or minimize sugars. As previously mentioned, starch and sugar discourage HCL production. In addition, sugars can initiate fermentation (Eaton 1991), which interferes with the ability of your pancreatic enzymes to digest your foods, and contributes to an unhealthy intestinal environment. Sugars provide an easy food for harmful yeasts, fungi, and bacteria (Matthews 1992), and the resultant microbial overgrowth is hard on your intestinal tract, and may trigger inflammation there (King and Toskes 1979).

Make every effort to eat at regular intervals. You may find (as many of us do) that your daily eating pattern is characterized by long periods where you can't or don't take the time to eat, followed by overeating when you finally do eat. In addition to stressing your digestive organs and your liver, this can contribute to blood sugar swings, which can hyperactivate and eventually exhaust your immune system. Over time, this can debilitate and deplete your whole body.

Some people have even reported that their blood sugar swings seem to correlate with their flare-ups.

Suggestions for Eating in Restaurants

Anyone who has rosacea knows that eating in a restaurant is always an adventure. "Did I remember to ask if the dish was spicy?" "Will they remember to leave out the tomatoes?" "Is there any chance I'll actually be able to eat everything or even anything on my plate?"

Well, as long as you're already engaged in a prolonged conversation with your waiter, you might as well make a few more requests and ensure that your meal is a healthful one and ultimately a well-digested one. If you're one of the many people with rosacea who seem to have digestive problems, try eating your protein first as suggested earlier in this chapter. To make this eating pattern easier, ask for your entrée first, so they won't wait until you finish the salad and bread before bringing you your main course.

You may notice that although your main course may seem fine, your vegetables or potatoes always seem to be loaded with pepper or some other spice you forgot to ask about. Remember, you can always ask for things to be cooked differently from how they are presented on the menu. Request that your vegetables be steamed rather than cooked in oil. Ask for the exact seasoning you want—a little salt, maybe a special herb. Not only is your food more healthful served this way, but, just as importantly, you will know exactly what you're eating. People with rosacea just hate those surprise ingredients. Do the same thing if you're offered a potato side dish. Ask for a baked potato, rather than something cooked in oil with seasonings you can't control.

Regardless of how careful you are, there are still pitfalls you may encounter in restaurant eating. Maureen, a sales rep for a cookware manufacturer, is a good example. Her job kept her on the road, which meant she had to eat in restaurants much of the time. She needed to keep her flares under control, because they affected her comfort level in dealing with customers. She tried to be really careful both in choosing her restaurants and in selecting "safe" foods that would also taste good and satisfy her. She went through a lot of trial and error and some very rough times trying to figure it all out:

"I have the most difficulty when I have to eat wherever the group I'm dealing with wants to eat. I finally figured out that as long as I avoided anything that had sugar, vinegar, tomato, chocolate, or MSG, I would do okay. So, I always asked for lemon and olive oil for my salads, and since the Chinese restaurants were usually pretty good ones, I was able to request no MSG. But sometimes, I would still feel my face start to flush, even though I knew I hadn't eaten any of these things. I couldn't figure out what was causing it. So I thought maybe I should dig a little further and find out if there was something else that I wasn't aware of that was somehow getting into the food. I have a territory I cover, and we usually end up going back to certain 'favorite' restaurants. So one time as I made the rounds, I decided to check out a few of the restaurants. I talked with the manager at some of them and was even able to talk with a number of chefs in some detail. It felt a little awkward and I was afraid my questioning would really be irritating. After all, no one else had any problems. But they were all really nice and I was glad I did it.

"Probably the most consistent thing I discovered, that I thought might be a problem, was that some of the restaurants were adding an onion flavoring to some of the dishes. It didn't seem a likely culprit, but I decided to see if this could be it. From that point on, at every restaurant, I asked them to please not use this onion flavoring or anything similar. Guess what? It made a difference. Later on one of the managers let me know that the onion flavoring had MSG in it. I finally had the answer to my flushing."

A good restaurant should be able to accommodate your needs. If something is not prepared the way you've requested, don't be afraid to send it back. Your skin and overall health require that you ask for what you need and that you get it.

Protectors and Enemies in Your Gut

Antibiotic users take note! The information that follows is especially important if you've been taking antibiotics. And if you have rosacea, the chances are slight that you've never had them prescribed for your face. Maybe you even stopped taking them because your digestive system started acting funny. Well, there's a reason you were in distress: When you take antibiotics, you kill off not only harmful bacteria throughout your body, but you also kill the beneficial bacteria in your intestinal tract. When the normal balance of bacteria is thrown off, the effects can seriously affect your digestion, which impacts your overall health. For this reason, it's important to consider taking probiotics if you have taken a course of antibiotics; it is so important to restore the beneficial flora. Probiotics come in capsule, powder, or even liquid form. A high-quality live-culture yogurt can also be helpful.

This section will introduce you to some critical players in your digestive process, usually ignored and poorly understood— your intestinal flora. Understanding your intestinal flora cannot be overrated, and keeping them in balance is absolutely crucial for your overall health, including the health of your skin. Let's take a look at how and why this is true.

First of all, would you believe that each of us has a good three pounds of flora (primarily bacteria and yeasts) in us—about the weight of our own liver? Not only do we have all these critters living in us, but we are also completely dependent upon them, in a symbiotic relationship, *without which we could not survive*. For purposes of general understanding, there are two overall categories of flora in your intestines: *beneficial* flora and *pathogenic* flora.

Your beneficial flora are wonderful. They help your digestive enzymes do their work and they also produce many essential nutrients for you, such as vitamins B_1, B_2, B_5, B_6, B_{12}, biotin, folic acid, plus vitamin K and even vitamin A. In addition, they produce certain other substances that actually serve as primary nutrients for the lining of your intestinal tract, particularly your colon.

Your pathogenic flora are another story. Anything that compromises the digestion of your foods provides a perfect environment for these "bad guys" to flourish. As you learned earlier, any circumstance that compromises Stage 1 of your protein digestion may seriously weaken the Stage 2 completion of protein digestion in your small intestine, leaving you with undigested and indigestible food in your small intestine. These undigested foods then provide a veritable banquet for your pathogenic flora, causing them to proliferate out of control and overwhelm your beneficial flora.

When these pathogenic organisms are engaged in their feast, they proliferate in your small intestine and create dozens, if not hundreds, of highly acidic and often caustic chemicals or toxins, known as "endotoxins." These endotoxins are the natural excretory waste of these pathogenic organisms (they are, after all, living organisms that eat and excrete). Dr. Joseph Pizzorno, a naturopathic physician, researcher, and founding president of Bastyr University in Washington, describes the havoc that results from this in his book, *Total Wellness* (1996, 112). Endotoxins can and do pass through the bowel wall into the body (Tagesson 1983) where they can damage enzymes and tissues (Roland et al. 1993) and cause disease (Belew et al. 1982). In addition, pathogens convert the breakdown products of food into toxic forms (Chadwick et al. 1992), and when pathogens die, their own breakdown products become additional endotoxins.

Dr. Jeffery Bland, Ph.D., a well-known nutritional biochemist, says, "These internally produced toxins must all be processed by the liver. If food is poorly digested, it can produce ammonia, alcohol, and other chemicals in the body as a result of increased putrefaction. The overgrowth of bacteria or yeast in the GI tract may create toxic overload that can stress detoxification" (Bland 1999).

Sugars and processed carbohydrates, which are nearly pure starch, can further complicate this process. Recall that fruits and refined starches require considerably less digestion time than proteins. When sugars and refined starches, which convert fairly quickly to sugar in your gut, are mixed in with concentrated protein, they cannot pass through and be digested at their usual pace. They can only pass through at the rate at which your protein food is processed. There they are, sitting in the warm, moist environment of your intestinal tract, like a dessert offering to the sugar-loving pathogenic yeasts and bacteria. Is it inconceivable that this would be a perfect environment for their fermentation activities? Add the excretions from these organisms to the ones generated by the protein-loving pathogens, and you have an "endotoxic" soup.

When your small intestine is in a healthy state, it is slightly alkaline. Yet when your food passes into your small intestine, it is very acidic. Because your pancreatic and small intestine enzymes require a more alkaline environment, your pancreas creates bicarbonate to neutralize the acid (Berne and Levy 1998). However, the excretions of both the protein-loving organisms and the sugar/

starch loving pathogens can force your small intestine to become increasingly acidic, which creates two major problems. One is that those specialized protein- and starch-digesting enzymes mentioned above are pH sensitive, and require the normally slightly alkaline environment to perform their functions. If the environment becomes too acidic, both the production and activity of these enzymes are compromised (Bland, Research/articles, case study). This may mean that more of your food is not thoroughly digested and therefore becomes available for the pathogens. In a way, the pathogens may be creating an environment that is favorable only to themselves.

The second major problem is that, while your pathogenic flora thrive under these conditions, your beneficial flora cannot tolerate such an acidic environment. They begin to die off, which means they produce less and less of their wonderful nutrients for you. This process affects not only your small intestine, but your colon as well, so that the beneficial flora that normally live in your colon also cannot thrive, and the pathogenic flora take over there as well.

With the intestinal flora out of balance, and the pathogenic flora having gained the upper hand, the extensive lymph tissue (vessels and nodes) embedded in your intestinal wall becomes activated. This is significant because the vast majority of lymph tissue in your entire body (figures range from over 50 percent to over 60 percent) resides in and around the walls of your intestinal tract (Lipski 2000). In fact, the intestinal tract, with its gut associated lymphoid tissue (GALT), has been called the largest immune organ in the body (Saputo 1999).

When harmful gut substances cannot all be eliminated by your intestinal immune tissues, the delicate lining of your intestinal tract can begin to erode from irritation and allow particles of partially digested food, and even some of the pathogens themselves, to pass through your intestinal wall. Once through the intestinal wall, they pass through a vein called the portal vein and head straight to your liver, where another big chunk (10 to 15 percent) of your immune tissue, known as Kupffer cells, resides.

Activation of the GALT, and subsequent activation of the Kupffer cells, can send a signal to the immune tissue in the rest of your body and can trigger a systemic alarm, leading to hyper-activation of your entire immune system.

Bland refers to this in the syllabus for the Fourth International Symposium on Functional Medicine. He reports, "The liver is known to sequester immunological fragments of antigen/antibody complexes that are delivered from the gut and can exert their effect on Kupffer cells in the liver. . . . the liver plays a principal role in communicating the message 'foreigner on board' from activation of GALT (gut associated lymphoid tissue). Activation of the Kupffer cells produces increased nitric oxide and oxidants, which can initiate liver-specific inflammation, as well as signal a pro-inflammatory state systemically" (233).

The condition in which food particles and pathogens pass through the intestinal wall is called intestinal permeability or "leaky gut," which we'll discuss in a bit more detail below. Your liver attempts to transform these harmful substances so that they can be excreted in your urine or stool. If the toxic load is too great and overwhelms the liver's capacities, whatever cannot be processed adequately by the liver passes into systemic circulation and has to be dealt with by immune tissues throughout the rest of your body. Over time, this constant load on your immune system is believed to debilitate and deplete your whole system (Lipski 2000).

Dr. Jeffry Anderson, M.D., a physician in environmental medicine in Marin County, California, corroborates this, reporting that "Recent research suggests that degradation of the gastrointestinal environment is one of the primary points at which health is lost. What we now know is that the same toxins associated with GI dysfunction are frequently absorbed and distributed to other parts of the body. First they place a burden on the liver and the immune system. If liver overload occurs, there will be spillover, and some of the toxins will be passed on to other organs or tissues" (1999, 125).

It is known that the largest organ of elimination is your skin, designed by nature to excrete bodily waste. In fact, it's been estimated that the skin eliminates more than a pound of waste per day. Given this, it becomes understandable that if you have an overload of toxins in your body, you might notice the effects of this on your skin.

Intestinal Permeability, a.k.a. Leaky Gut

Some researchers think leaky gut is a major source of systemic inflammation. Apparently it can either *lead* to food sensitivities or can be the *result* of food sensitivities (Percival 1997; Lipski 2000). In his book, *Power Healing* (1997), Dr. Leo Galland, M.D. says, "excessive permeability permits excess absorption of antigens and microbial fragments from the gut, overstimulating the immune response, fostering allergy and autoimmunity" (205). He further states that symptoms produced by excessive intestinal permeability can include fatigue, joint and muscle pain, headache, and skin eruptions, and that the clinical disorders associated with increased intestinal permeability include any inflammation of the large or small intestine, chronic arthritis, and skin conditions like acne, eczema, hives, or psoriasis, etc. In his book, *Total Wellness*, Dr. Pizzorno says, "The problem with bowel toxins becomes even worse when the intestinal mucosal barrier becomes damaged. Not only does this allow more toxins to enter, but it also allows the entry of viable bacteria, pieces of dead bacteria and yeasts, and dietary proteins. This results in a huge overload for the liver. It also results in food allergies" (113).

Does Leaky Gut Have Implications for Rosacea?

The term leaky gut has begun filtering down to the general public, and a number of people have been questioning whether it could be a factor in their rosacea outbreaks. The following is a case history that may show this question to be truly worth considering:

Steve, an attorney in Grand Rapids, was treated for a year for what his internist thought was adult acne. When it didn't get any better, and in fact got worse with treatment, Steve went to a dermatologist and was diagnosed with rosacea. He then followed the standard rosacea treatment regime. However, as time went on, his condition got worse, and he found himself getting pretty depressed. He was put back on antibiotics when his flare-ups got out of hand, but he was getting worried because he didn't feel good on them, and it seemed like he was taking them more and more often. He also gained some weight, and to top it off, felt his energy level waning. Finally, depleted physically and emotionally by his struggle with rosacea, he went to a physician who specialized in natural medicine. The doctor took an extensive health history, asking Steve questions about his heritage, his food intake, and especially his digestion. Before they were finished, the doctor said he suspected Steve might be dealing with a condition called leaky gut. Steve looked at him incredulously, thinking for a minute that maybe it was a joke. The doctor laughed and explained what it was and that it might make sense, given Steve's symptoms and history, to test for it.

He described how the test, called the lactulose/mannitol test, measures the degree of intestinal permeability in the small intestine (Furlong 1999). He explained to Steve that he would be asked to drink a solution containing two special types of sugar, lactulose and mannitol, that are totally benign and that are not able to be broken down in the intestinal tract. After a period of time, a urine specimen would be collected to check on their absorption through his intestinal wall. Mannitol molecules are fairly small, and a healthy intestinal wall would allow it to be easily absorbed. However, lactulose molecules are much larger and would not be absorbed unless the intestinal wall had become too permeable. Therefore a healthy test result would show a high level of mannitol and a low level of lactulose in the urine.

Steve's test came back showing a large amount of both mannitol and lactulose in his urine, which is a marker for leaky gut. At first this seemed unnerving to Steve, but the doctor knew exactly what to do. First of all, he commended Steve for his efforts in avoiding the standard rosacea trigger foods. He also asked him to cut back and eventually eliminate sugar, including juices and dried fruit. Rather than jumping into a lot of additional testing, which Steve did not want to do, the doctor recommended that Steve eliminate gluten grains like wheat, rye, oats, barley, kamut, and spelt, and that he also avoid soy. The suggested diet was very simple: He was to eat mostly lightly cooked vegetables, fish (but not shellfish), poultry, rice, and fresh fruits. The doctor also had him get some cod liver oil capsules and flax seed (to grind and store in his freezer). To help heal Steve's intestinal lining, he recommended:

* Cod liver oil — 2 caps twice a day

* Flaxmeal — 1 to 2 tablespoons a day

* L-glutamine — 1000 mg twice a day between meals

* Quercetin chalcone — 250 mg twice a day

* Phosphatidyl choline complex — 1200g 3 times a day

✳ Evening primrose oil   500 mg 3 times a day
                                          with meals.

He also asked Steve to keep bottled water with him throughout
the day, and drink about six 8-ounce servings a day between
meals.

After about three weeks, Steve went back for another visit to
review his progress. His face hadn't shown much change, but it
hadn't gotten any worse either. He was feeling better, had more
energy, and had lost some weight. He also reported that he was
sleeping better. He was advised to continue on the program, and
to add some good olive oil to his diet if he liked. He was also put
on a good probiotic to help reinoculate his intestinal tract with
beneficial flora. He was asked to take only a small amount at first
and then build up to a larger amount, to make sure his system
received it well.

After about three months, Steve was feeling great. He had
his old energy back, and his rosacea flare-ups were considerably
reduced in both intensity and number. He told the doctor he felt
like he had a new lease on life.

Perhaps there is a relationship, one that we are just beginning to discover, between what happens in that mysterious chan-
nel that runs right through the center of us, our GI tract, and what
happens on our face.

IO

The Psychology of Face

By now you have a pretty good idea of how to interpret your triggers, as well as some new knowledge about how to treat your skin from the inside and out. However, your brain is actually your best ally in dealing with rosacea—and the next several chapters will focus on this all-important organ and how it relates to and influences the way we perceive our faces and our self-worth.

One instinct that we have from birth is the ability to recognize a human face, and the ability to recognize what human features are supposed to look like. For instance, when newborns are shown a simple circle (representing a rudimentary human head) with simple dots, dashes, and curves for eyes, nose, and smiling lips, it makes them happy. But if you present a Picasso-type head, with both eyes on the same side of the nose, babies will cry. It seems, then, as if they are preprogrammed to bond with the archetype of face.

To further emphasize its importance, the face is the only part of the body that contains all five senses: ears, eyes, nose, mouth, and the ability to feel tactile stimulation. No wonder it's regarded as the "headquarters" of the entire body.

Identity

If the eyes are the windows of the soul, then it must follow that the face is its front wall. It's not accidental that your face is regularly the first part of your body that you look at in the mirror. And it's a little paradoxical that it is also the only part of the front of your body that you need a mirror to view.

Your face is a handy way for society to recognize, categorize, characterize, and maybe even criminalize you. Do you want to drive a car? Your photo will be laminated onto your license. Fancy a trip to a foreign country? Not without your face emblazoned on a passport. A danger to society? Quick, unsmiling mug shots are the first stage of locking you up.

Society quickly discovered that your face "gives you away" or allows you to be recognized most easily. Are you a famous movie star, hoping for a few hours of peace as you do your grocery shopping? Changing your customary high heels for a pair of sneakers isn't quite going to do it. But wearing shades and thus altering your face will work most of the time.

Perhaps, you'll argue, fingerprints or DNA are more accurate. Maybe you're right. But could you pick out your own DNA or fingerprint profile from a group of twenty? Highly doubtful. Could you pick out your own photo from a group of twenty? Every time.

And therein lies the rub. You identify so closely with your face that when it changes quickly, due to an accident or a disease, it freaks you out. It is disturbing to have a stranger look out at you from your very own mirror. You are a sophisticated version of the newborn, wrestling with a messed-up configuration of the features you had grown to love and expect. Now you are no longer who you used to be. The world is no longer a safe place. If you can't trust your own face, how can you trust anything? You are being morphed before your very eyes—and the result is a psychological earthquake.

Throughout human history, people have used masks to hide from themselves and from others, but also to liberate hidden qualities within themselves. Shamanistic societies used masks (especially animal masks) in dance and ritual to symbolize and actualize the energies and characteristics of the depths of the psyche. Even in modern societies, the masked ball has permitted people to try out aspects of personality or forbidden behavior that would be unthinkable if one were "barefaced."

In ancient Greece, the actor had an array of masks from which to choose before he came on stage. The mask he appeared in was a *clue* to the audience as to what type of character it might expect. In Greek, the word for mask is "prosopon." The Romans translated this as "persona" (per-sonat, literally "that through which sound comes"). From this come the words "person" and "personality." So "personality" really is the mask you wear in order to clue the "audience" as to what kind of character it may expect. The ability to wear different masks is vital. Getting identified with a single mask leads to psychological atrophy. And a change of face may well be an invitation to a change of heart.

Character

There is native wisdom that claims a person's character can be inferred from their face. This tradition claims that while one may wear one's heart on one's sleeve, the face is the real giveaway. Not only does each human emotion tend to rearrange the face in a highly particular way, such that a trained observer can tell from a still photo what emotion the subject is feeling; but, more deadly still, face is thought to betray excessive indulgences—the wrinkled skin of the habitual smoker, the swollen face and puffy eyes of the heavy drinker, the vacant stare of the drug addict, or the narrow, cunning eyes of the lecher. It's a very handy system, and it's completely wrong. It's simplistic and it assumes guilt until innocence is proven. Perhaps the wrinkled skin belongs to an avid gardener who spent years in the sun. Perhaps the swollen face and puffy eyes belongs to a chronically allergic individual. That's why there are such well-known adages as "never judge a book by its cover." And yet, there was even at one period a psychology subspecialty that claimed to be able to accurately judge the character from the face. It was called *physiognomy*.

Many innocent people throughout history have suffered greatly at the hands of simplistic profiling that stereotyped their physical attributes according to some cultural fad. The fashion queens of exotic countries (e.g., the "fat and shiny" beauties of Nigeria, the huge-butted Hottentots of South Africa, or the long-necked women of Burma) would be a curiosity or even a laughingstock in the modern West. Conversely, the emaciated, pale-skinned wannabe fashion models of the West would be objects of pity or fear (they'd be taken for ghosts) in Papua New Guinea.

Though beauty may, indeed, be merely skin deep, the judgment is, frequently, that it indicates an unblemished character. And the opposite, unfortunately, is equally true. Facial blemishes of various kinds are frequently misinterpreted as indicators of unhealthy or even depraved lifestyles. It's bad enough to have a disease that disfigures the face, but to bear the extra burden of watching the beholder turn away in embarrassment, fear, or disgust is truly a heavy load. It takes a really mature and evolved soul to wear a diseased face without covering it over with either shame or anger.

Perception

Even an ordinary conversation can be traumatic if you identify yourself as a "rosacea sufferer." It becomes easy to assume that when people are looking at you as you speak together, they are not really seeing you but examining your "bumps" and redness. On the other hand, if they don't look at you during a conversation, you may presume it's because your disease embarrasses them. So you're damned if they do and damned if they don't.

If you chance upon someone whom you believe to be psychic, your reaction may be "Oh, no! She sees into my soul. She knows my darkest secret." It's not a very comfortable situation. But with a facial disease such as rosacea, you don't have to be in the company of a psychic, seer, or prophet to feel that your darkest secret is exposed. You are wearing it right up front. You may as well have the scarlet letter or the number 666 tattooed on your forehead. It's there for even the most unsophisticated or casual observer to notice and judge.

It's relatively easy, then, to feel misunderstood and misperceived. You feel as if people will think your condition is due to either bad habits or poor hygiene. It is a terrible burden to have to carry. And the salt in the wound is that, physiologically, the shame or anger at being misunderstood worsens the situation by flooding the facial blood vessels, thus initiating a vicious circle of disease → symptoms → perceived judgment by others → reaction in the psyche → escalation of symptoms. Is it all bad news? No, it definitely is not. It is quite informative to study demographically matched pairs, each one of whom is similar in background, age, socioeconomic status, ethnicity, educational level, and symptomology, and then run a battery of psychological tests. What happens is that from nearly identical profiles you can have very different outcomes, because one member of the pair has been crushed by the disease, while the other member has transcended it. And what is the deciding factor? Read on.

Reframing

There are several theories of emotion in the psychological literature. One theory suggests: stimulus → emotional response →
physiological reaction. In this theory, you come around a corner
in the shrubbery and come face-to-face with a hungry man-eating
tiger (the stimulus). This leads to a feeling of intense fear (the
emotional response). The fear provokes a whole set of bodily
reactions: your pupils dilate, hair stands up on the back of your
neck, blood abandons your body's surface (making you feel cold)
and concentrates in the muscles (getting you ready for fight or
flight, to be either a gladiator or an Olympic sprinter). This is the
physiological reaction.

A second theory of emotion suggests a different progression:
stimulus → physiological reaction → emotional response. In this
model, the sight of the tiger leads first to the bodily reactions, and
it is these bodily reactions that trigger the emotional response.
Subtle difference, same outcome: tiger flossing teeth after a great
meal.

A third theory of emotion adds an extra and vitally important fourth element. In this scenario you come around the corner
of the same, by now well-trodden path, and there before you is
the man-eating tiger (occasionally known to also feast on females)
staring you in the face. This time you think, "Wow, what a mag-
nificent creature!" as you watch the exquisitely muscled torso,
mystical eyes, long tail, and superb coat. Thereupon follow the
emotional response and physiological reaction in any order you
choose. Unlikely scenario, says you. You're off your rocker, says
you. Who in their right mind is going to admire a man-eating
tiger? Well, there is one important detail that needs to be added.
In this third pass, the tiger is in a cage in the zoo, and you have
gone there specifically to see him. So you came around a corner
from the hippos and the monkeys and there he was. Cheap trick,
you say. No, not at all—it's precisely the point. This third theory
posits that there is a quick cognitive element between the stimulus and the emotional/physiological piece. And it is that flash of
interpretation that determines if and what the emotional/physio-
logical piece is going to look like.

So if the corner around which you strolled was in a jungle in
India with nary a cage nor a McDonald's in sight, the mental
interpretation would very likely be, "I'm in deep serious trouble
here." In such circumstances, nobody would complain of your

body odor if you chose to sweat profusely, or call you a wimp if you attempted a sub-four-minute mile. If, however, the corner around which you walked so jauntily was at a traveling circus, and that same striped feline were to eye you hypnotically, your future offspring would not hold you accountable for dallying a while.

The mental interpretation is the all-important missing link. However, it happens so fast that even psychologists at first missed it. But once they got it, they went on to develop a healing tool from it. They called it "reframing," or choosing to consciously make a better interpretation of a stimulus. For example, in a phobia, an objectively neutral stimulus such as an elevator can cause great fear, even panic or catatonia. At some level, a cognitive distortion has conferred terrifying properties on the little mobile room. Reframing would be a way of seeing the elevator as a friend that saves your legs and wind as you attempt to visit your ninety-three-year-old, asthmatic grandmother on the forty- third floor.

What of reframing and rosacea? No doubt by now you have put together, consciously and unconsciously, a host of associations and interpretations about your appearance, how you are perceived, your prognosis, and your self-worth. Many of these are the result of lightning-quick mental judgments. The very good news is that the easiest part of the psyche to change is the thinking. One good lecture, one great teacher, one fortuitous book can forever change what you believe about yourself. Emotional beliefs follow on a little more slowly.

You remember the "little engine that could"? Well, it's true. You can change your mind—literally. Every new idea lays down a new configuration of neuronal connections in the brain. As a result, embedded belief systems about rosacea and its impact on your life imprint on your physical brain a pattern of associations between the cells. For example, if you permit people to walk across your lawn, pretty soon they're going to pound out a grassless track. In order to revitalize your lawn, you have to prevent them from walking through it and insist they walk around it. The brain is like that. A long-held idea beats out a path in the brain. To eradicate such an idea, you have to stop using it and develop a new idea. This is what happens in reframing. And when you're finally able to do this, your reality changes. Then you will find that your perspective about the importance of this disorder in your life will also change. Reframing will be discussed further in the next chapter.

II

Everything You Can Have

It's really no fun having any kind of disorder. Yet you may sometimes feel guilty being so unhappy about something that is "just
your skin." Even people close to you may ridicule you for your
concern. But the fact is that most illnesses are not out there for the
world to see. If you have irritable bowel syndrome, no stranger
on the street is aware of it. If your body aches, the person you're
doing business with is most likely oblivious to it. But your face—
now that is a different matter. Unless you take to wearing a veil,
it seems like everyone can see what kind of day you're having.
The following chart, based on surveys by the National Rosacea
Society, shows the emotional fallout of rosacea. But it's important
to add that when rosacea symptoms improve, emotional health
also improves.

Rosacea can be emotionally very painful. You may find
yourself constantly looking in the mirror, dismayed that your
complexion is doing this to you. However, you need to keep
reminding yourself that, as with most things in life, you notice
much more about yourself than other people do.

Think about it: How many times have you heard friends
complain about some terrible flaw in their appearance that you've
never even noticed? In reality, the feature that bothers you most
will hardly register with others. Or if it does, they don't really
give it much thought. They see it and then move on to worrying

Rosacea's Impact On Daily Life

Rosacea sufferers feel:

Low self-esteem

	75%

Embarrassed

	70%

Frustrated

	69%

Robbed of pleasure/happiness

	56%

about their own expanding hips or their too fat belly or perhaps those new lines and wrinkles. We have a tendency to forget how self-involved people can be, especially about physical appearance. People around you just don't spend a lot of time thinking about how you look.

You will also notice, as time passes, that a blotch or a flush that once would have made you frantic suddenly doesn't seem quite as important. It's as if the mind adjusts and no longer demands perfection. It's one of the healthiest things that can happen to you—and it's amazingly liberating. Just keep in mind that even if it hasn't happened to you yet, it eventually will.

The most important thing of all is to avoid letting rosacea control your life. It's not easy, because it's a disease that initially presents so many limitations, so many things you can't have, so many things you can't do. This sense that everything is the enemy can be just overwhelming. By rosacea's very nature, it almost forces you to be constantly aware of it. And in itself, that feeling of perpetually being on guard causes considerable stress. And stress, as you well know, is a primary trigger. So around and around you go.

Changing Your Perspective

However, there is a way out of this harmful mind-set. Like so much in life that hinders you, it can and must be reframed, as discussed in the previous chapter. The way you probably deal with rosacea is to note your triggers—everything that is now closed off to you. If you're like most people, you focus on all the things that make you different and separate you from your friends and family and life as you once lived it.

But you can turn this around. Instead of making mental or written notes of everything you can't eat, start listing everything you can eat. Instead of thinking about all the activities you can't enjoy, start thinking about slight modifications that will allow you to continue those activities. And to make your life more interesting, start adding brand-new activities and adventures to it.

Rosacea is not life-threatening. You know you're not going to find yourself rushed to the emergency room because of an attack of papules and pustules, so you can't let it limit your enjoyment of life.

Look Around You

Let's look at this logically. For example, if you're a typical rosacea person, you're always complaining about everything you can't eat. But take that thought further and realize how very limited your food selection was even before you were diagnosed. How often did the food in your refrigerator vary? How many different things did you cook? Look at menus in restaurants and realize that you've seen and eaten the same items over and over again, year after year. Boring, isn't it?

Are you starting to realize that the reason your food choices are limited now is that they were so limited to begin with? Like everything else in life, you've started with such a small sample that once you've eliminated a few things, it seems like a major loss.

The sensible thing, then, is to make your sample much larger. To do this, you must expand your food choices. Start by asking yourself some simple questions. How many types of fruit have you ever eaten? How many vegetables? How many different grains are you familiar with? Do you realize how many ethnic cuisines are eaten in America alone? How many have you ever tried? There's more to American cuisine than Chinese, Thai, and Italian food.

There's literally a world of food choices out there for you. Experiment and try at least one new thing a week. Think about the joy of making eating fun again. If you have a reaction, so be it. Try something else. Your options will amaze you.

Make Adaptations

Chances are that you have been curtailing activities that you once loved. Maybe you've stopped going to cafes with your friends. Start doing it again, because you can still drink coffee or tea. Just let it cool down, or have it iced.

If you want to hike, you should do it, and do it regularly. Exercise is vital for your physical and psychological well-being. Just choose a time of day when you can avoid full sunlight, bring cold water, and of course, wear a sunblock and a hat that shades your face. Early morning or late afternoon is a wonderful time to be outside. Better yet, find places that are shaded where you can hang out any time of day. And if you flush a little, you flush. You'll survive it. The important thing is that you're out there again, enjoying your life.

Experiment! Be creative! Marie just hated the idea of giving up her hot tub, which had always been one of her greatest joys in life. She was determined to occasionally still use it. So, when she feels her rosacea is under good control, she gets in the tub after lowering the temperature to warm instead of hot. She then sucks on ice chips while in the tub, and also sprays her face with cold water. In the summer, she lowers the heat to body temperature or less and uses the tub as a way of cooling down.

Marie is also addicted to her exercise bike. She has found two tricks that help cut way down on overheating and subsequent flushing: using a fan and sucking on ice chips. She is determined not to let rosacea rob her of all the things that she loves to do.

Anne, an exercise enthusiast, was determined to keep up with the aerobics program to which she had been devoted for years. Before rosacea, she was a runner; now she is an avid swimmer, swimming at least a mile a day. She has also discovered water aerobics, which she loves. "Not only don't I flush anymore during exercise, but the water program is so much better on my joints than running ever was. I don't consider this as something in place of running anymore—it's really exactly what I want to be doing." Anne adds a useful tip: "I always make sure to wash the chlorine off my face if I'm in a pool or the salt off my face if I swim in the ocean. I've learned the benefit of that firsthand."

Remember that there are a great many things you **can** do. Think of rosacea as an opportunity to expand your life, rather than as something that limits it. Once you put this spin on it, you'll immediately see it lose its control over you. Take some time now to think of all the new experiences you're going to have.

With Change Comes Growth

With rosacea, you're forced to deal with every aspect of your life, because every aspect of your life affects rosacea. The paradox is that the thing that you regarded as the problem has the potential

---

"Things I <u>Can</u> Have"

New foods to try

Foods I can eat

Old activities I like to do and new ways to do them

New activities to try

---

to become the springboard for extraordinary personal growth. The "triggers" of rosacea, so long seen as a limiting force in your life, can instead be viewed as triggers to change your life. Rosacea can make you more creative in all areas, from the way you eat to the way you fill up your day, and, most importantly, in the way you perceive yourself.

Problems cause change, and not just on a personal level. In the history of the evolution of our planet, every quantum leap has been triggered by some global crisis. One interesting example: The first sea creatures evolved about 700 million years ago, but they encountered a problem. The very seawater they needed for their survival contained so much calcium that by metabolizing it, they were taking in toxic quantities. They needed to deal with the excess. Their first response was to become garbage collectors, dumping vast quantities of calcium, which gave us the great coral reefs. Millennia later, they came up with a more creative response: They built domiciles out of the extra calcium. These were the first crustaceans. This solved the problem and also afforded them protection. A third and even more creative response was to interiorize the extra calcium in the form of a skeletal system. This, in turn, gave them great mobility and strength.

The whole purpose of problems is not that they simply beg solutions, but that they afford the possibility of self-transcendence. Psychologists say that the presenting symptom or crisis is often the gateway to a much more comprehensive addressing of deeper issues. For many, rosacea is such a crisis. So make use of it and let it be a springboard to realizing your full potential.

Michael is a good example of this principle. He made the choice to use his personal crisis in a positive way. "I was always just an average kind of guy, living a pretty boring life. I wasn't involved in much of anything. When I got rosacea, I just holed up in my apartment for a few years feeling sorry for myself. Then one day, it suddenly occurred to me that life is very short, and I was missing it. When I got honest with myself, I realized that I had been missing out on life long before I had rosacea. Since eating in restaurants was always difficult, I started to prepare my own meals. I got so good at it that I became a gourmet cook. Realizing that stress was a huge element in causing my face to flare, I learned about meditation and visualization. Then I got into deep breathing and journaling. All this has led to an exponential increase in my ability to relax in all areas of my life. I never thought I'd say this, but for me, I'm glad I developed rosacea.

Working with it has made me much more outgoing and relaxed in business and in my personal life."

Exercise: Transforming Crisis

Think of a situation in which an illness or crisis proved to have been the best thing that ever happened to you or someone close to you.

Example: Johnny was an eighteen-year-old high school senior with a great future as a football player. However, he had a serious drinking problem and wouldn't listen to anyone about it. One night while drinking, he had an automobile accident and broke both legs. Luckily, no one else was hurt. Johnny missed the first semester of college, and his career as a football "star" was over—and he knew it was because of the alcohol. Today he is a thirty-five-year-old football coach who says that he truly believes that the accident saved his life. "I have a good life now and I enjoy my work. After the accident, I was forced to deal with my drinking. If that hadn't happened, it's not inconceivable that the next time behind the wheel I could have killed myself or some innocent person on the road."

Now it's your turn:

Education

There is one more thing you can do if you're willing, and that's educate people around you about rosacea. If you put yourself out there and tell "your audience" about rosacea, the results are twofold. First, letting people know that the blemish on one's face is not a blemish on one's character, turns ignorance and prejudice into knowledge and understanding. This is a very valuable service to perform for those people who have no idea what rosacea is all about. If someone is staring at you, it's only because they're curious. Talk to them. If you're uncomfortable in front of your coworkers, then talk to them too. Explain that you have a very common, noncontagious skin disorder. The benefit to you is that explaining to people what you're experiencing will help you relax, and your level of discomfort will diminish dramatically. Telling people what is real about rosacea strengthens your own positive self-image, because it allows you to rest in the security of being seen for who you really are.

And what you'll find out is that people are really interested in learning about the existence of rosacea. They'll probably tell you that now that they think about it, they've seen it a lot, perhaps in their own family, or even in their own mirror. They just never understood what they were seeing before.

Will, a grocery store employee, says he got annoyed and embarrassed because a coworker kept staring at his red, slightly swollen nose. Finally, Will just told him that it was due to rosacea. The coworker was very interested and wanted to know all about it. Will says, "The funny thing is that I actually gave him a gift. He had been convinced that his father, a recovered alcoholic, was secretly drinking because his nose had developed a similar appearance. It was a tremendous relief for him to know that his father just had rosacea, and also a relief for his father to know what was happening to his face."

The more you tell the same story, the more you're convinced of its reality. If your tendency is to emphasize the limitations of rosacea, your life becomes limited. If you choose to turn it around and see rosacea as presenting opportunities to expand your life, that's what will happen. It's as simple as that.

12

Face It, You're Not Your Face

When you first develop rosacea, all your time and energy go into thinking about everything that now appears to be off-limits to you. It seems like a terrible curse that is destined to curtail your enjoyment of life. But by now we hope you are learning to view it differently—to realize that fate now demands that you see rosacea not as the focus of your life, but as just a part of your life. And, in truth, actually not a very important part.

Taking Back Your Life

There are ways to take away rosacea's power to control you. For example, how many times a day do you look in the mirror—six times, a dozen, two dozen or more? What does this behavior accomplish, except to make you crazy? You can't let the quality of your day be determined solely by the state of your complexion. With rosacea, there are times when your face seems to change by the hour, if not by the minute. If you allow your mood to be tied in to how you look at the moment, you will spend each day on an emotional roller coaster. Realize that constantly peering at yourself is as unhealthy for you as going on and off the scale is for someone with an eating disorder. It is compulsive, harmful behavior.

At first, you'll have to consciously restrain yourself from mirror gazing. Actually writing down how many times a day you look at yourself will give you a good idea of your level of fixation. Set an upper limit for the day and see if you can keep to it. Once you've succeeded, great, reduce the number even further. Gradually it will get easier, and you'll find that scrutinizing yourself becomes less important to you. At that point, you should only be using the mirror when necessary, such as when applying some product to your face, or in order to ensure that your eyeliner actually ends up in the general vicinity of your eye.

Eat the foods that you thrive on, enjoying the fact that you've actually expanded your choices. Take your time and don't worry about a reaction. Assume that you will be fine. Make mealtimes a pleasure again, rather than a time of worry and stress. Take your nutrients every day with the idea that you're doing it for your entire well-being, both physical and emotional. Don't think of it in terms of something you're doing just for the rosacea. Do everything you do with a focus on benefiting your whole being. Taking the emphasis off the rosacea is a way to loosen its power over your life.

Rosacea may be the initial catalyst for you to adopt stress-reducing techniques, but ultimately it will improve all areas of your life. Learning to control stress is a gift that doesn't recognize the boundaries of particular illnesses, but benefits the entire physiology and psychology of a person. Make stress reduction a part of your daily routine. Again, not because you have rosacea, but because, as for everyone else, it's beneficial to your health. Find the technique that works for you. It may be that sitting quietly and breathing deeply does the trick, or you may be drawn to different types of meditation. Meditation is particularly helpful because it is the most ancient way of disidentifying with ego. To help you realize that you are not just your face.

There are support groups on the Internet that can be very helpful, especially in the beginning when you have so many questions about rosacea. A lot of useful information can be shared in this way. It's also comforting to find a group that shares your concerns. However, at a certain point, you should think about limiting your participation in these groups. It keeps you too focused on rosacea when you're constantly reading about it and thinking about it. Somebody writes about some weird reaction they're having to water and all of a sudden you have it too. Why do you think medical students suppose they have every disease they read about? Because they're immersed in it. Don't make that mistake. Don't make rosacea your life.

Rosacea is just something on your face. You will ultimately decide how much it will limit you. It is important for you to look out through your eyes at the world and not at the mirror. Concentrate instead on what interests you about life. There is a present and a future in that for you, but there is neither in the mirror.

You can end rosacea's control over you in one of two ways. The first way is to do the best that you can for the condition and then, finally, just relax with it. You've realized that you're just tired of it all. You decide that enough is enough, and that you want to fully participate in life. You don't want it passing you by anymore. The second way is to find an inspirational system that allows you to reframe the importance of one physical attribute, which is all rosacea really is.

Exercise: Seeing the Real You

Conversion or recovery is never so much a question of turning away from one viewpoint or practice, but rather the turning toward an alternative viewpoint or practice. Try a simple exercise. List what you appreciate about yourself in the following categories:

Physically

For example: I like the color of my hair.
I like the length of my fingers.
I like the fact that I'm physically fit.

Now fill in your own list:

Emotionally

For example: I like the fact that I'm a patient person.
I appreciate that I don't hold grudges.
I like that I can genuinely feel happy for other
people's successes.

Now fill in your own list:

_____

_____

_____

_____

Intellectually

For example: I like the fact that I'm a curious person.
I appreciate that I like to think deeply.
I like that I can locate the geographical names
in a newscast.

Now fill in your own list :

_____

_____

_____

_____

Spiritually

For example: I like the fact that I'm a compassionate person.
I appreciate the awesomeness of nature.
I find great peace in my meditation.

Now fill in your own list:

_____

_____

_____

_____

Now list what you like about yourself in relationship with others:

For example: I like that I'm a loyal friend.

I like that I can overlook my friends' foibles.

I like the fact that I remember people's birthdays.

Now fill in your own list:

_____

_____

_____

_____

_____

Realize that these are the characteristics that are core to who you are—much more than the appearance of your skin. After all, you have never lost a real friend because of your rosacea. Even if physical appearance is initially either an impediment or an attraction, very quickly true friendship begins to be built on a deeper appreciation of the other.

Therapy

Everyone should be able to identify characteristics that they admire in themselves. If either a childhood experience or a reaction to an illness has such traumatic consequences that your self-image consists only of negatives, then you need to seek professional help. A therapist can help you identify the origins of this misperception and help you rebuild your self-esteem.

Even if your self-perception hasn't fallen quite that low, dealing with rosacea may have depleted your internal resources. If that's the case, therapy should also be considered.

The Choice Is Yours

Rosacea symptoms can vary considerably from one person to another. For some they're mild, for others more severe. But ultimately the decision is the same for everyone. To live your life fully, rosacea has to be put in the background. It can happen sooner or it can happen later, but it has to happen. You will reach an age when you realize that it's not worth caring about any more. Life has a way of doing that to us when it concerns physical attributes. Chances are that aside from your rosacea, you are a reasonably healthy person. Take advantage of that, throw away your mirror, and go out into the world and enjoy your life.

Appendix

Insurance Coverage for Rosacea Treatments

The chronic nature of rosacea and its current invulnerability to any permanent cure can make it an expensive disease to treat. The ameliorative treatments that are available, such as reconstructive surgery for rhinophyma cases, laser and PhotoDerm, and other treatments that have been described previously in this book, are costly.

In an age of cost containment, a rosacea patient and her treating physician can be confronted with an uncooperative insurer. It is difficult to generalize about the exclusions or policies that lead to denial of coverage by a health insurer because of the vast array of insuring arrangements that provide coverage for Americans. The law applying to ERISA, HMO coverage, preferred provider coverage, group coverage, individual policies, and other arrangements differs from case to case. The language of the policies, the exclusions that apply, the law of the insurance code for a specific state, all come into play when a decision is made by the insurer whether to cover a given treatment for rosacea.

In the course of writing this book, we used Internet chat rooms to conduct an informal poll among rosacea patients about this subject. The successes and failures of people who contacted us mirrored the confusing welter of laws and policies listed above. Some were reimbursed by insurers for the cost of laser, photoderm, and other treatments. Others were met with a flat "no" by their insurance company. An important factor did seem to be the extent to which the treating physician was willing to go to bat for the patient and to make a strong case for the treatment in question.

The possibility of insurance coverage for rosacea treatment, however, should not be overlooked or dismissed out of hand. Informal consultation with lawyers familiar with insurance coverage questions led us to the conclusion that there are rarely any "bright lines" that indicate whether treatment for a disease like rosacea will be covered or not, and quite often the decision will be made on a case-by-case basis.

As a starting point for understanding this issue, we note that an insurance company attempting to deny coverage for a rosacea treatment often takes the position that the treatment is "elective" or "cosmetic" and not "medically necessary" or a "medical necessity." The latter test is often applied in deciding whether to extend coverage for an ameliorative treatment, and this general language is often found in insuring agreements or group benefit plans. For example, a patient seeking coverage for breast augmentation might be denied coverage on the ground that such surgery is "cosmetic" and not "medically necessary"; a post-mastectomy patient might be covered for very similar surgery on the ground that it is reconstructive.

Such an example may suggest to the rosacea patient that a decision regarding coverage has a large subjective component regarding "medical necessity," and this viewpoint finds a great deal of support in the legal cases that have decided coverage questions.

As an example specific to rosacea, a person with severe rhinophyma may find himself stigmatized as an alcoholic or suffer debilitating social and occupational consequences. These consequences could in turn lead to psychological problems such as depression. Curiously, many insurance policies would probably cover the costs of psychotherapy on the ground that ameliorating depression is a "medical necessity" and in some cases, even a matter of life or death. The question then arises: Why should the treatment of the *root cause* of the loss of self-esteem and depression be denied coverage as "cosmetic" or "elective"? These distinctions again suggest the arbitrary way in which coverage decisions for rosacea treatment (and other dermatological treatments) are made.

Treatments for other symptoms of rosacea differ from the rhinophyma example only by degree. Rosacea sufferers can attest to the negative life consequences of flushing, acneiform lesions, and other symptoms. These manifestations of the disease certainly can rival the disfiguring effects of burns and other skin conditions which may be insurable for reconstructive therapies. To deny coverage for one type of problem on the ground that it arises from a "disease," and to cover another but no worse disfigurement because it involves a skin graft or scar revision may not make sense on the ground that one is "cosmetic" and the other is "medically necessary."

These comments are offered as general guidelines in seeking coverage. The language of a given policy or benefits handbook should always be consulted to determine the wording of exclusions and the conditions and treatments that are insurable. As mentioned, these vary from contract to contract. Other factors certainly come into play when the rosacea patient consults with her physician about seeking coverage. For example, will there be an effect on premiums? Is there a problem with preexisting conditions? If the treatment is justified because of the psychological problems associated with the symptoms, will this disclosure have negative repercussions elsewhere in the patient's life? In an age where medical records seem to be increasingly in the public domain for all kinds of review, this latter consideration will of course be important.

Where medical treatment for rosacea is important and potentially effective, however, and the patient is inadequately funded for the treatment without coverage, a careful consultation with a physician and submission of a proposed plan of treatment to the insurer should definitely be considered. Rosacea patients *do* receive insurance benefits for treatment in some cases. Denial of coverage under one plan or contract does not rule out the possibility of coverage under another plan with different conditions and terms.

References

Aloi, F., C. Tomasini, E. Soro, and M. Pippione. 2000. The clinicopathologic spectrum of rhinophyma. *Journal of the American Academy of Dermatology* 42:468-472.

Anderson, S., M. Rosenbaum, J. Bland, et al. 1999. The Basics. In *Optimal Digestion*, edited by Trent Nichols and Nancy Faass. New York: Avon Books.

Anderson, J. 1999. How problems with digestion can cause illness anywhere in the body. In *Optimal Digestion*, edited by Trent Nichols and Nancy Faass. New York: Avon Books.

Balch, J.F., and P. Balch. 1997. *Prescription for Nutritional Healing. Second Edition.* Garden City Park, N.Y.: Avery Publishing Group.

Belew, P.W., E.W. Rosenberg, R.B. Skinner, et al. 1982. Endotoxemia in psoriasis. *Archives of Dermatology*, 118:142-43.

Berne, R.M., and M. Levy. 1998. *Physiology. Fourth Edition.* St. Louis, Mo.: Mosby, Inc.

Bland, J. 1999. Toxic Overload. In *Optimal Digestion*, edited by Trent Nichols and Nancy Faass. New York: Avon Books, Inc.

———. 1997. Fourth International Symposium on Functional Medicine, syllabus. The Institute for Functional Medicine, Aspen, Colorado May 15–17, 1997.

————. Digestion, enzymes, and nutrient absorption. Research Article for Nutritional Counseling Six: Practice Management and Ethics Case Studies, p.RA-5.

Borrie, P. 1953. Rosacea with special reference to its ocular manifestations. *British Journal of Ophthalmology* 65:458.

Cabot, S. 1999. *The Healthy Liver & Bowel Book.* Berkeley, Calif.: Celestial Arts.

Chadwick, R.W., S.E. George, and L.D. Claxton. 1992. Role of the gastrointestinal mucosa and microflora in the bioactivation of dietary and encironmental mutagens or carcinogens. *Drug Metabolism Review,* 24:425-492.

Clinical Pearls. 1997. Clinical Pearls interview with U.N. Das, M.D., FAMS, FICN, FICP, Chief of Division of Internal Medicine, Clinical Immunology and Biochemistry L.V. Prasad Eye Institute Banjara Hills, Road #2 Hyderabad-500 034 India. referencing his clinical report entitled, "Oxidant Stress, Anti-Oxidants and Essential Fatty Acids in Systemic Lupus Erythematosus, Mohan, I.K. and Das, U.N. Prostaglandins, Leukotrienes and Essential Fatty Acids, 1997:56(3):193–198.

Crayhon, R. 1994. *Nutrition Made Simple.* New York: M. Evans and Company.

DeVries, C.E. and C.I. Van Noorden. 1992. Effects of dietary fatty acid composition on tumor growth and metastasis. *Anticancer Research.* 12(5):1513-1522.

Eaton, K.K. 1991. Gut Fermentation: a reappraisal of an old clinical condition, diagnostic tests and management—a discussion paper. *Journal of the Royal Society of Medicine* 11:669-671.

Enig, M. 2000. *Know Your Fats.* Silver Spring, Md.: Bethesda Press.

Fallon, S., and M. Enig. 1999. *Nourishing Traditions.* Washington, D.C.: New Trends Publishing.

Furlong, J. 1999. How to find out what's working and what isn't. In *Optimal Digestion,* edited by Trent Nichols and Nancy Faass. New York: Avon Books.

Gaby, A. 1997. Sesame seeds for high blood pressure. *Nutrition & Healing.* October.

Galland, L. 1997. *Power Healing.* New York: Renaissance Workshops, Ltd., Random House.

Gerster, H. 1998. Can adults adequately convert a-linolenic acid (18:3n-3) to eicosapentaenoic acid (20:5n-3) and docosahexaenoic acid (22:6n-3)? *International Journal of Vitamin Nutrition Research* 68:159-173.

Gittleman, A. 1999. *How to Stay Young and Healthy in a Toxic World*. Los Angeles, Calif.: Keats Publishing.

Gottschall, E. 1997. *Breaking the Vicious Cycle*. Kirkton, Ontario: The Kirkton Press.

Golan, R. 1995. *Optimal Wellness*. New York: Ballantine Books.

Grant, J., and J. Joice. 1987. *Food Combining for Health*. Rochester, Vt.: Thorsons Publishers.

Halberg, L., et al. 1987. Phytates and the inhibitory effect of bran on iron absorption in man. *American Journal of Clinical Nutrition* 45:988-96.

Hitch, J.M. 1967. Acneform eruptions induced by drugs and chemicals. *JAMA* 200:879-80.

Holmes, P. 1994. *The Energetics of Western Herbs. Revised Second Edition*. 2 vols. Berkeley, Calif.: NatTrop Publishing.

Jenkins, M.S., S.I. Brown, S.L. Lempert, and R.J. Weinberg. 1980. Ocular rosacea. In *Ocular Therapeutics* by B.D. Srinivasan. New York: Masson Publishing.

Keville, K. 1995. Anthocyanidins and proanthocyanidins. *The Herb Report*. The American Herb Association 11:3.

King, E., and P.P. Toskes. 1979. Small intestine bacterial overgrowth. *Gastroenterology* 76:1035-1055.

Krohn, J. 1991. *The Whole Way to Allergy Relief and Prevention: A Doctor's Complete Guide to Treatment and Self-Care*. Point Roberts, Wash.: Hartley & Marks, Inc.

Kunin, R. 1999. Nutrients for repair. In *Optimal Digestion*, edited by Trent Nichols and Nancy Faass. New York: Avon Books.

Lalles, J.P., and G. Peltre. 1996. Biochemical features of grain legume allergens in humans and animals. *Nutritional Review* 54(4):101-107.

Lininger, S., J. Wright, D. Brown, S. Austin, and A. Gaby. 1998. *The Natural Pharmacy*. Rocklin, Calif.: Prima Publishing.

Lipski, E. 2000. *Digestive Wellness. Updated Second Edition*. Los Angeles, Calif.: Keats Publishing.

Marinkovich, V. 2000. Phone interview with Donna Shoemaker on July 12, with Dr. Marinkovich's verbal approval for inclusion of this information.

————. 1999. Taped interview with Jeffery Bland from transcript of *Functional Medicine Update*. Gig Harbor, Wash.: HealthComm, Intl. November.

Matthews, G. 1992. Gut fermentation. *Journal of the Royal Society of Medicine* 85:305.

Mercola, J. M. 1999. Ulcer bacteria treatment helps rosacea. *Townsend Letter for Doctors & Patients*. June.

Mindell, E. L. 1997. *The MSM Miracle—Enhance Your Health with Organic Sulfur*. New Canaan, Conn.: Keats Publishing, Inc.

Murray, M., and J. Pizzorno. 1998. *Encyclopedia of Natural Medicine, Revised Second Edition*. Rocklin, Calif.: Prima Health, a division of Prima Publishing.

Murray, M. 1996. *Encyclopedia of Nutritional Supplements*. Rocklin, Calif.: Prima Publishing.

Noguchi, M. 1995. The role of fatty acids in eicosanoid synthesis inhibitors in breast cancer. *Oncology* 52:265-271.

Nolan, J.P. 1989. Intestinal endotoxins as mediators of hepatic injury—an idea whose time has come again. *Hepatology* 10: 887–891.

National Rosacea Society. 1998. *Coping with Rosacea* (pamphlet).

National Rosacea Society. 1997. *Rosacea: What You Should Know* (pamphlet).

National Rosacea Society survey. 1999. *Feature 2.* (survey) *Rosacea Review.* Fall

O'Laoire, S. 1997. An experimental study of the effects of distant, intercessary prayer on self-esteem, anxiety, and depression. *Journal of Alternative Therapies* 3(6):38-53. November.

Pederson, M. 1994. *Nutritional Herbology, A Reference Guide to Herbs*. Warsaw, Ind.: Wendell A. Whitman Co.

Percival, M. 1997. Nutritional support for detoxification, in *Clinical Nutrition Insights*. San Clemente, Calif.: Advanced Nutrition Publications, Inc.

Pizzorno, J. 1996. *Total Wellness*. Rocklin, Calif.: Prima Publishing.

Rateaver, B., and G. Rateaver. 1973. *The Organic Method Primer*. Pauma Valley, Calif.: self-published.

Reinhold, J. G. 1972. Phytic acid combines with Fe (iron), Ca (calcium), P (phosphorus), and Zn (zinc) in the intestinal tract so that these minerals cannot be absorbed. *Ecology of Food and Nutrition* I:187-192.

The Rodale Institute Study. 1997. A comparison of corn/soybean cropping systems under conventional management for 15 years, reported in "Organic Farming Improves Soil Quality." *Delicious* 12/97, 16.

Roland, N., L. Nugon-Baudon, and S. Rabot. 1993. Interactions between the intestinal flora and xenobiotic metabolizing enzymes and their health consequences. *Wrokd Rev. Nutr. Diet* 74:123-148.

Salyers, A.A. 1979. Energy sources of major intestinal fermentative anaerobes. *American Journal of Clinical Nutrition* 32:158-163.

Saputo, L. 1999. Harmful flora. In *Optimal Digestion*, edited by Trent Nichols and Nancy Faass. New York: Avon Books.

Schmid, R. F. 1987. *Traditional Foods Are Your Best Medicine*. New York: Ballantine Books.

Schmidt, M. 1997. *Smart Fats: How Dietary Fats and Oils Affect Mental, Physical and Emotional Intelligence*. Berkeley, Calif.: Frog, Ltd., distributed by North Atlantic Books.

Stahl, W., U. Heinrich, H. Jungmann, H. Sies, and H. Tronnier. 2000. Carotenoids and carotenoids plus vitamin E protect against ultraviolet light-induced erythema in humans. *American Journal of Clinical Nutrition* 71:795-798.

Tagesson, C., et al. 1983. Passages of molecules through the wall of the intestinal tract. *Scandinavian Journal of Gastroenterology* 18:481-486.

Tubaro A., et al. 1984. Evaluation of anti-inflammatory activity of a chamomile extract after topical application. *Planta Medica* 50:359.

Timmons, W. 1999. *Assessing GI Function, GI Gluten/Food Profile* (audio taped seminar). San Diego, Calif.: BioHealth Diagnostics.

Werbach, Melvyn R. 1996. *Nutritional Influences on Illness. Second Edition*. Tanzana: Calif.: Third Line Press.

Wilkin, Jonathan. 1999. National Rosacea Society. Rosacea Review. Winter.

Zand, Janet, and Allan Spreen. 1999. *Smart Medicine for Healthier Living*. Garden City Park, N.Y.: Avery Publishing Group.

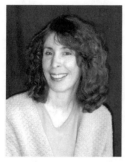

Arlen Brownstein, M.S., N.D., is a Naturopathic Physician and also has a masters degree in nutrition from the University of Connecticut. As a sufferer of rosacea and as an ND, Dr. Brownstein has researched its triggers and treatment for the past eight years.

Photo by Sharon Thom

Donna Shoemaker, C.N., is a Certified Nutritionist and nutritional counselor, researcher, and health educator practicing in Marin County, California. She received her BA from the University of Michigan and her Certified Nutritionist degree from American Health Sciences University. Donna's background includes hospital and social service work, as well as organic farming and gardening.

Sean O'Laoire, Ph.D., is a clinical psychologist and a Catholic priest in the San Francisco Bay Area.

Some Other
New Harbinger Titles

The Woman's Book of Sleep, Item WBS $14.95

The Trigger Point Therapy Workbook, Item TPTW $19.95

Fibromyalgia and Chronic Myofascial Pain Syndrome, second edition, Item FMS2 $19.95

Kill the Craving, Item KC $18.95

Rosacea, Item ROSA $13.95

Thinking Pregnant, Item TKPG $13.95

Shy Bladder Syndrome, Item SBDS $13.95

Help for Hairpullers, Item HFHP $13.95

Coping with Chronic Fatigue Syndrome, Item CFS $13.95

The Stop Smoking Workbook, Item SMOK $17.95

Multiple Chemical Sensitivity, Item MCS $16.95

Breaking the Bonds of Irritable Bowel Syndrome, Item IBS $14.95

Parkinson's Disease and the Art of Moving, Item PARK $16.95

The Addiction Workbook, Item AWB $18.95

The Interstitial Cystitis Survival Guide, Item ICS $15.95

Illness and the Art of Creative Self-Expression, Item EXPR $13.95

Don't Leave it to Chance, Item GMBL $13.95

The Chronic Pain Control Workbook, 2nd edition, Item PN2 $19.95

Perimenopause, 2nd edition, Item PER2 $16.95

The Family Recovery Guide, Item FAMG $15.95

Healthy Baby, Toxic World, Item BABY $15.95

I'll Take Care of You, Item CARE $12.95

Call **toll free, 1-800-748-6273,** or log on to our online bookstore at **www.newharbinger.com** to order. Have your Visa or Mastercard number ready. Or send a check for the titles you want to New Harbinger Publications, Inc., 5674 Shattuck Ave., Oakland, CA 94609. Include $4.50 for the first book and 75¢ for each additional book, to cover shipping and handling. (California residents please include appropriate sales tax.) Allow two to five weeks for delivery.

Prices subject to change without notice.